In today's age where n   th, it is
important that we under   al health,
and spiritual health should be equally prioritized. Dr. Vetere is
able to weave these together in a digestible way so they can be
accomplished and maintained.

—ALLAN HOUSTON
CEO, ALLAN HOUSTON ENTERPRISES
FORMER NBA ALL-STAR

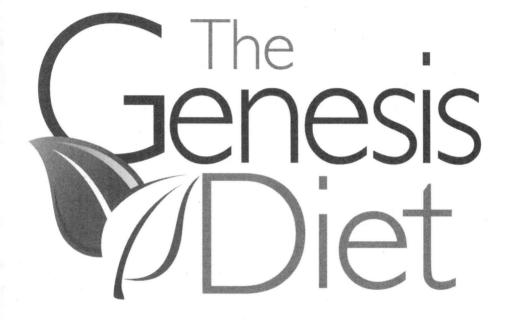

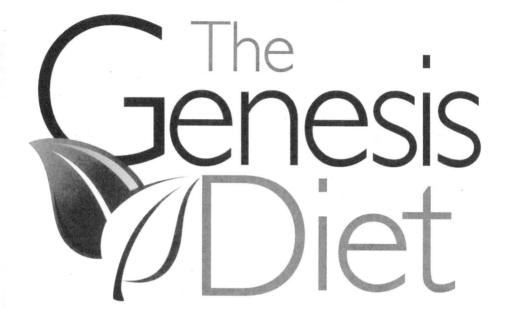

The Genesis Diet

JOSEPH VETERE, DC

SILOAM

Most CHARISMA HOUSE BOOK GROUP products are available at special quantity discounts for bulk purchase for sales promotions, premiums, fundraising, and educational needs. For details, write Charisma House Book Group, 600 Rinehart Road, Lake Mary, Florida 32746, or telephone (407) 333-0600.

THE GENESIS DIET by Joseph Vetere, DC
Published by Siloam
Charisma Media/Charisma House Book Group
600 Rinehart Road
Lake Mary, Florida 32746
www.charismahouse.com

Unless otherwise noted, all scripture quotations are from the New American Standard Bible, copyright © 1960, 1962, 1963, 1968, 1971, 1972, 1973, 1975, 1977, 1995 by The Lockman Foundation. Used by permission. (www.Lockman .org)

Scripture quotations marked KJV are from the King James Version of the Bible.

Cover design by Justin Evans
Design Director: Bill Johnson

Visit the author's website at http://www.schoolofwellness.com.

Library of Congress Cataloging-in-Publication Data

Vetere, Joseph.
The Genesis diet / Joseph Vetere.
    p. cm.
Includes bibliographical references.

ISBN 978-1-61638-495-1 (trade paper) -- ISBN 978-1-61638-701-3 (e-book) 1. Health. 2. Weight loss. 3. Christians--Health and hygiene. I. Title.
RA776.5.V48 2012
613.2'5--dc23

2011037524

12 13 14 15 16 — 987654321
Printed in the United States of America

This book is dedicated to all those who have tried everything to get in shape but have yet to taste success: Know this...the Lord and His Word are unfailing. He has a plan for your health and well-being!

CONTENTS

ACKNOWLEDGMENTS

THE WRITING OF this book must be credited to the thousands of patients over the past twenty-five years who have entrusted me with their health and wellness. So a special thanks to all the patients who give me purpose and joy, those who challenge me, and even those who question me and cause me to grow.

Thank you to...

- That extraordinary group of praying patients who have encouraged me through the process, whose feedback and kind compliments were always refreshing

- My precious wife for putting up with the long hours and long stories that go along with the running of a health center and for her unwavering support in all my endeavors

- My daughters, who continuously remind me that they are my greatest fans

I want to give special thanks to Alice Bocachica, whose decades of prayers and encouragement were priceless. And thank you to...

- Tony Cavallo for his steadfast support in both the valleys and on the mountains

- My business partner, Dr. Robert Reiss, who after twenty-five years still thinks I have great ideas

- My "Genesis Life" team for their hard work and long hours

- My brother Mike and his wife, Deidre; Lissette; Pete; and my cousin Carlo

A special thanks goes to Debbie Marrie, who saw this book as a great idea before I wrote chapter one, and Carol Noe, my editor, for her faithful expertise.

And finally I want to thank my pastor, Glenn Harvison, who always has my back, and my mentor, Dr. Myles Munroe, who always has the time to pour a powerful Word into my life.

FOREWORD

T HIS ERUDITE, ELOQUENT, and immensely thought-provoking work gets to the heart of the deepest passions and aspirations of the human heart: *longevity*. The desire for extended, healthy life is the twenty-first century's obsession. The health lifestyle industry generates billion of dollars, and yet many have not found the success they pursue.

The Genesis Diet is a profound authoritative work that spans the wisdom of the ages and yet breaks new ground in its approach and will possibly become a classic in this and the next generation. It is indispensable reading for anyone who wants to live life above the norm and rediscover the oldest wisdom on health that is still valid for today.

I found this exceptional work by Dr. Joseph Vetere to be one of the most profound, practical, principle-centered approaches to the subject of health that I have read in a long time. The author's approach to this timely issue brings a fresh breath of air that captivates the heart, engages the mind, and inspires the spirit of the reader to understand and embrace the powerful principles of health found in the oldest document on the earth.

The author's ability to leap over complicated theological and metaphysical jargon and reduce complex theories to simple practical principles that the least among us can understand and apply is amazing.

This work will challenge the intellectual while embracing the layman as it dismantles the mysteries of our soul-search for good health and long life; it delivers the profound in simplicity.

Dr. Vetere's approach awakens in the reader the untapped inhibitors that retard our personal physical development and health habits; his anecdotes empower us to rise above these self-defeating, self-limiting factors to live a life of exploits in spiritual, mental, and physical advancement.

He also integrates into each chapter the time-tested precepts of biblical wisdom, giving each principle a practical application to life and making the entire process people-friendly.

Every sentence of this book is pregnant with wisdom, and I enjoyed the mind-expanding experience of its exciting message. I admonish you to plunge into this ocean of knowledge and watch your life change for the better as you rediscover and experience the life and health the Creator intended for you—from the genesis of life.

—DR. MYLES MUNROE
BAHAMAS FAITH MINISTRIES INTERNATIONAL FELLOWSHIP
INTERNATIONAL THIRD WORLD LEADERS ASSOCIATION
NASSAU, BAHAMAS

INTRODUCTION

I REMEMBER WORKING WITH my marketing team to create a promotional ad for an upcoming healthy lifestyle workshop. The pastor who was hosting the event was really into fitness himself. He was excited to have his congregation challenged in the area of personal wellness. He told me that a lot of people in the church needed to lose weight, and he wanted me to put something in the flyer to catch their attention, something that would really spark their interest.

I had just recorded a CD called *How to Lose a Pound of Body Fat Every Three Days*. I decided to make that the headline for the workshop. It worked. The place was packed with people who wanted to see if what I said was true or just another diet "hype."

Their comments were insightful. "Wow, that sounds great! I would love to lose a pound of body fat every three days. But is it true? Can that really be possible?" Others proposed: "There has to be some catch to it. Probably an impossible-to-do-diet and workout routine required." Some even wondered astutely, "Is it scientifically possible to lose weight and body fat at such a fast rate?"

The truth is that not only is it possible, but also some people can actually lose more body fat at a greater rate than what I suggested. It's not about a crazy restrictive diet plan or spending hours on the treadmill. The key to making it happen is *simply positioning yourself for success and taking ownership of healthy lifestyle actions.*

WHY SOME PATIENTS GET WELL WHILE OTHERS DON'T

I have observed in my twenty-five-plus years of chiropractic practice that some patients get well and achieve their healthy lifestyle goals while others don't. In pondering the reason for the lack of success for some, I have analyzed the differences between patients who are successful and those who are not.

In certain cases, the severity and the longevity of the health condition overwhelm the patient's hopes for success. In most situations, however, the difference is simply an improper positioning of the patient because of faulty mental, emotional, or spiritual issues. For example, many just want to be given a pill or five easy steps to losing weight or accomplishing other health goals.

From my professional observation, wellness is most often achieved by embracing proper mental, emotional, and spiritual positioning. The patients who do not succeed in reaching their health goals were not willing or able to make the real-life adjustments that would assure their success. These adjustments need to occur before a patient is able to develop any *repetitive and sustainable positive healthy lifestyle habits.*

If you're the type of person who says, "Just show me the formula for losing the fat; I don't care about all this positioning and behavior modification," you will most likely remain among the ranks of millions of people who try program after program but never achieve lasting success in their health goals.

In working with thousands of patients over the years, I have learned that it is more important to resolve in your mind and heart the "why I should get healthy and lose weight" issue rather than the "How do I lose the weight?" question. Unfortunately, most people just want to jump right to the how-to part of getting into shape. Their approach is: "Tell me what to eat." "What exercises should I do?" "How long will it take?" But this mentality usually ends in a fleeting commitment to diet and exercise followed by a sense of failure, which eventually gives way to a "Why bother anyway?" attitude.

Getting into shape, losing weight and body fat, and achieving optimal health and wellness naturally must begin with a rock-solid mental, emotional, and spiritual positioning regarding the underlying issue: "Why I should be healthy." Taking ownership of this vital issue in your heart is the only way to succeed in exercising the habits that govern good health, persistently and continuously.

You see, if your goal is just to lose weight at any cost, there is a good chance that you

> Wellness is most often achieved by embracing proper mental, emotional, and spiritual positioning.

may engage in activities that could compromise your overall wellness. Diet pills, weight-loss shakes, and crash diets may all help you to lose unwanted pounds. But these fad regimens may also cause you to lose your health in the long term. The side effects of the medications or even so-called "natural caffeine"–laden products can cause severe and irreversible damage to organs and glands. As for crash diets, while you may lose a few quick pounds, these regimens are completely unsustainable. They rob your energy, tax your immune system, and eventually result in rebound weight gain that is greater than your original weight.

Your goal should be *wellness* rather than *weight loss.* As a matter of fact, weight loss is inevitably the end result of establishing good lifestyle habits to achieve wellness. Working on your wellness means you're improving your overall health. Not only will you decrease your chance of becoming a victim of major illness, but you will also gain vitality, increase your energy levels, and, of course, reach your ideal weight.

A SPECIAL PICTURE OF GOD'S DIVINE PLAN

> Then God said, "Let Us make man in Our image, according to Our likeness; and let them rule over the fish of the sea and over the birds of the sky and over the cattle and over all the earth, and over every creeping thing that creeps on the earth."
> —GENESIS 1:26

The special picture of the design and plan God had for mankind revealed in this scripture has been a life motivation for me. Made in the likeness of God and given dominion over our surroundings, we were intended to enjoy abundant life, developing the attributes and characteristics of God and living in fellowship with Him.

Working on your overall wellness may seem to be a loftier objective than just losing weight. But to me, according to the Scriptures, pursuing overall wellness fits in better with the grand scheme of God's plan for your life. I believe that from God's perspective, while achieving your ideal weight would be nice, to experience optimal health would be even better. His perfect design for mankind was all-inclusive for the benefit of living life as He ordained it to be.

WHY FOCUS ON THE BODY FAT FACTOR?

Since we are not born with the perfect design God intended, I realize that you have to start somewhere. My purpose for presenting the concept of losing body fat quickly is not just to get your attention; it is intended to give you opportunity to understand the foundation for the science of getting into great shape. Addressing hidden spiritual and psychological issues will help to position you for success in achieving your health goals.

Simply stated, *The Genesis Diet* is much more than a simple way to eat; it is a recipe (diet) for healthy living in every area—spirit, soul, and body.

So why should you focus on losing body fat? Isn't that the same concept as losing weight? Not exactly. You may be aware that the concept of losing body fat is based on a group of contributing factors that coincide with lifestyle habits governing overall wellness. The numerical loss of body fat pounds (body fat percentage) are markers used by physicians to track wellness progress and to direct fitness habits.

Your ideal body fat percentage cannot be achieved by simply losing weight. It is achieved primarily through correct eating habits, including appropriate nutritional intake, along with a proper balance of aerobic, strength, power, and endurance exercises. In addition, you can't dismiss the necessity for drinking plenty of water, getting adequate rest, eliminating harmful stress, and insuring a properly functioning nervous system. These are some the positioning factors we will discuss that will assure your success in your long-term wellness goals.

OBESITY IN THE UNITED STATES

- The latest statistics say that 68 percent of Americans are overweight and 34 percent are considered clinically obese.[1]

- According to the US Census Bureau, there were 308,745,538 American citizens in 2010.[2] That would mean 210 million Americans are overweight and 105 million are clinically obese.

- Latest studies released by the National Bureau of Economic Research indicate that the medical cost associated with obesity is well over $168 billion annually.[3]

- These studies also suggest that obesity adds $2,800 per person annually to their medical costs over people who are not obese.[4]

- If that is not enough, clinically obese people have an increased risk of cancer, diabetes, and heart disease.

These statistics are shocking for two reasons. First, the epidemic of obesity is almost completely *avoidable*. This is a crisis born out of poor choices and terrible lifestyle habits. Scores of people are unnecessarily getting sick and dying prematurely of diseases that could be prevented by avoiding obesity. In addition to the tragic loss of quality of life and life itself, the economic loss is staggering; that is, unless you are in an ownership position of a hospital, a health insurance company, or a pharmaceutical company. Businesses like these profit from our poor lifestyle choices.

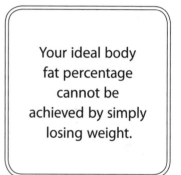

Your ideal body fat percentage cannot be achieved by simply losing weight.

Secondly, these statistics are shocking to me personally, as a believer in the gospel of Christ, because Christians understand that their body is the "temple of the Holy Spirit" (1 Cor. 6:19). While Christians confess that God the Holy Spirit dwells in them, they cultivate destructive eating habits, hate to exercise, and create tons of self-induced stress, much like non-Christians.

As Christians, we believe in a God who is Jehovah Rapha (the Lord Our Healer) and a Savior who is the Great Physician. Yet I have treated many Christian patients who are sometimes in worse shape than their non-Christian counterparts. Our churches are filled with overweight and obese children and adults who are unwittingly circumventing the grace of God for their health through poor personal lifestyle choices.

It seems we do not understand, as born-again believers, that we do not have a special immunity to sickness just because we are Christians. Though we may give up bad habits such as smoking, drinking, and so forth, if we do not follow biblical principles for caring for our temple, we will suffer the same consequences to our health as our non-Christian friends do.

THE PURPOSE OF THIS HEALTH PROTOCOL

The primary goal is to get you to your ideal body fat by improving your overall wellness. To do that, I will introduce you to scientifically sound principles that align as well with timeless biblical covenants. These powerful biblical principles reveal God's design and plan for living the abundant life through establishing a healthy lifestyle—body, mind, and spirit.

The overriding purpose for guiding you to your ideal physical prowess will be to give glory to God, your Creator—not for your personal vanity. Getting into great shape and attaining optimal health by means of obedience to divine precepts of biblical covenants will not only let you live the abundant life they promise, but it will also make you an effectual witness in the earth to the truth that our God is still in the healing business.

> We do not have a special immunity to sickness just because we are Christians.

Chapter 1

THE *WHY* IS MORE IMPORTANT
THAN THE *HOW*

I**N MANY SELF-HELP** books the major premise revolves around the how-to concept. People who buy a self-help book hope to discover five easy steps that will tell them how to achieve their desired goals. Though authors sincerely want to help their readers learn the *how-to* for getting the help they need, there is a larger issue that many books do not address. That is the *why* they should pursue specific health goals.

Can the intentional hype necessary for book sales be misleading? Are authors addressing the underlying issues that may sabotage the reader's ability to reach their goals? Can the reader be successful simply by complying with the how-to steps taught in the book? My experience in working with thousands of patients who have read these books tells me otherwise.

> The primary goal is to get you to your ideal body fat by improving your overall wellness.

I have personally read dozens of fabulous motivational books for a healthy lifestyle written by highly qualified authors. I have marveled at their breakthrough science, brilliant concepts for dietary habits, and ingenious exercise methods that are cutting edge in the world of fitness. Then, in consulting with my patients, I ask them if they have read these books. They have. So I wonder why they are in my office. Didn't they get what they read? Why didn't they follow through with what was taught in the books?

Finally it dawned on me. We have developed into a society of people who pride themselves in looking for shortcuts. People open a self-help book, flip through the table of contents, and go right to the chapter on "How to…" Just show me what to do right now! It better be quick, easy, and painless. If the title of the book is *5 Steps to Lose*, the prospective reader may perceive instead: *5 Easy, Quick, and Painless Steps to Lose.*

Don't get me wrong; it is imperative to have an easy-to-understand, scientifically sound how-to methodology for any successful self-help book. That is especially true with books that deal with improving one's health. But is giving people the how-to enough to make the reader compliant to the lessons presented? Again, my experience with patients tells me, "Not at all."

CONSIDERING THE IMPORTANT *WHY* FACTOR

For years I studied my patients to try to understand the answer to this vital question: Why do some patients achieve their health goals while others do not? I do my best to explain to each of my patients the procedures and methods that have proven to be successful to establishing a healthy lifestyle. Some patients follow through with these methods; some don't. As I analyzed the motivation of my patients, I found a consistent difference between those who succeeded and those who did not.

My successful patients have one thing in common: their profound understanding of *why* they should be well is greater than their desire for a shortcut way of *how to* get well. Their clear and persuasive understanding for why they should be well makes them considerably more compliant and goal oriented than patients who do not succeed in reaching their health goals.

The specific goal for your health presented in this book is to get you to your ideal body fat percentage and help you achieve optimal natural wellness. I will show you step by step exactly how to reach those goals. But to assure your success, there are issues that must be addressed, which could otherwise hinder you from reaching your fitness goals. The first is to develop a clear, persuasive argument that you can own in your heart for *why* you should get yourself into shape: *Why* should you follow the necessary how-to section of this book?

In summary, getting into shape, losing weight and body fat, and achieving optimal health and wellness must begin with a rock-solid mental, emotional, and spiritual positioning regarding the underlying issue: why I should be healthy. Taking ownership of this vital issue in your heart is the only way to succeed in exercising the habits that govern good health, persistently and continuously.

THREE DIFFERENT MOTIVATIONS
FOR PURSUING HEALTH

Over the years I have noticed three reasons why people are motivated to lose weight, eat better, and improve their lifestyle habits. One of the reasons relates only to temporary success, one may be too late, and only one results in permanent and life-transforming success.

Time-sensitive vanity

The first reason people become motivated to lose weight is because of what I call *time-sensitive vanity*. There's a wedding coming up or a class reunion, and you want to show up looking good, like you're really in great shape. This motive is prideful and very shallow, not exactly attributes of a Christian. Don't get me wrong when I say that I partially approve of this faulty motivation. It can become a great adjunct in the support or initiation of lifetime success, a starting point to take you forward into a healthy lifestyle.

I encourage you to look good *all* the time so you feel good about yourself all the time—not only physically but also mentally and emotionally as well. The better you view yourself physically, the less self-conscious you become and the more confident you are. Looking good draws attention to the lifestyle changes you have made; it gives you an opportunity to witness to what you have done and share the plan you have followed.

The problem is, if the motivation is just for the temporary goal date alone, what happens after that date is passed? Do you go back to the old habits that kept you out of shape in the first place? Probably. Without positioning yourself in the right mind-set emotionally, mentally, and spiritually for lifetime success, cookies and doughnuts will be right back on the menu.

There is another serious problem with this prideful, shallow motivation. Time-sensitive vanity is usually more *time sensitive* than the person realizes. They want to lose twenty-five pounds or drop five dress sizes in a few months. Unfortunately, there is no safe health plan that can pull that off. So these people may resort to unnatural or risky methods for weight loss that can cause more harm than help. Time-sensitive vanity goals are only good when they don't make you vain and they motivate you continually for special events throughout the year. That means you set goals that you want to look good for your birthday, Christmas, and the Fourth of July party, so you follow a healthy lifestyle consistently to that end.

Facing a health crisis

The next reason many people choose to lose weight and get into shape is based on desperation. They are not just focused on losing body fat; they are trying to save their life. This motivation is the one that I cited as probably coming too late. It is precipitated by *crisis*.

You may be twenty-five pounds overweight and have a body fat of 38 percent (3 percent above the clinical obesity line). But you feel relatively fine and have no urgent health concerns. More than likely you are not going to race to my office and knock down my door for an appointment. Nor are you going to stay up all night reading this book in one sitting to find answers you don't feel you need.

What happens in more than 90 percent of people is that they live a complacent life, slowly and steadily getting out of shape. Every year they get a little bigger and move a little slower. They take a few more mild medications to keep what they consider minor health conditions under control. They settle for a lifestyle of mediocre wellness instead of the Lord's promised abundant life; then the day of the crisis arrives.

Suddenly the pain in the chest is intense, they suffer shortness of breath, and they are startled by the yellow color of their eyes. They never expected that they would have to call 911 for help—or that the matter of their life or death would be in the hands of an overworked EMT who would rush them to an emergency room where an even more overworked and underpaid doctor was attempting to save their life. They never considered that maybe the ambulance would not get to their house on time because of traffic or that the emergency room doctor was really an exhausted resident in training with seven months of experience.

If, by the grace of God, they survive, they suddenly become motivated to pursue a healthier lifestyle. "Yes, Dr. Vetere, tell me what to eat and I'll do it; show me the exercises, and I'll be at the gym every day; eight glasses of water a day, eight hours of sleep every night, no more coffee, no more soda. I'll be at your office every day for my spinal adjustments; I'll even wash your car for you."

While crisis may be the *great motivator,* it is definitely not the *best* motivator. The problem with crisis-based motivation, though very effective in getting your attention, is that quite often the damage is already done.

The ability to regain your God-ordained vitality is gone after suffering that damage to your body.

You may ask, "Can't God create a complete healing?" Of course He can. I don't doubt anything regarding what God can do or what God will do. But the point I am making is that most crisis-related disorders never had to be a crisis in the first place. I believe that good health is a blessing based on our obedience to the laws of God regarding His design for the body and His covenants (precepts) that govern wellness.

Break the covenants and suffer the consequences. Get your lifestyle in alignment with principles that dictate good health, and your restoration will be forthcoming. After experiencing a crisis, you can only hope that you last long enough for complete healing to occur. For my part, I believe in youthfulness at any age and vibrancy every day I live as I choose to consistently obey divine principles for a healthy lifestyle.

Especially for the crisis-motivated person, being aware of the body fat percentage health marker is the ideal approach to health. In my experience, people who are motivated to change as a result of crisis can sometimes go overboard in their efforts, trying to regain everything they lost in their health crisis overnight. Instead, they should make it their objective to develop a plan for regaining health, one that is safe and practical. Learning to evaluate their body fat percentage and other health markers and working to improve it consistently is a safe plan for everyone and is especially effective for the crisis-motivated person.

Again, the keys to being successful, whether your goal is to lose twenty pounds of body fat, naturally reduce your blood pressure, or just get into better shape, is to mentally, emotionally, and spiritually position yourself for lasting success. (See chapter 2.) In large part, that vital positioning is the result of embracing the *why* of your pursuit of optimal health.

Exercising wisdom

The third reason people are motivated to achieve optimal health goals is by far the most sensible and categorically the least practiced. I call it *exercising wisdom*. We have all heard the adage, "Knowledge is power." That may be true, partially. But I believe that it is in *applying* knowledge that it becomes true power. *Wisdom* may be defined, according to Webster, as "good judgment, insight, and a wise attitude or course of action"[1]—in other words, *applied knowledge.*

The truth is that you can have all the knowledge in the world, but if you don't have the wisdom to apply that knowledge, it becomes ineffective. Here's my (slightly biased) best example of knowledge without wisdom. Medical doctors, nurses, and other allopathic-related practitioners all have the knowledge of how the body works; they know the risks of poor lifestyle habits. But there is little evidence that these health care providers are any healthier than the general population.

On the other hand, most chiropractors, naturopaths, and holistic nutritionists I know personally are in significantly better shape than the general population (my biased opinion based on my interaction in the profession). Why? Well, by example, they have to practice what they preach, or no one will accept their healing methods.

In fact, many holistic healing professionals, who embrace New Age philosophies, deny the lordship of Christ and some even the existence of God. Yet they are in better health, suffer less chronic disease, and live life more abundantly than some Christians. You might wonder how they inherited the promises made to faithful followers of Christ. The answer is simple. They applied the knowledge of the divine principles that govern the ability of the body to maintain health. Admittedly, some of their practices may be far-fetched and unscientific, which we must reject entirely. But those practices are simply a ploy of the enemy to keep Christians away from the sensible and scientific practices offered through natural health care.

The point is that your obedience to the biblical principles that govern health will result in good health, whether you have faith or not. Wisdom, which is applied knowledge, works for everyone who practices its principles. If you want to attain your ideal body fat percentage, lose weight, get rid of aches and pains, or naturally resolve your diabetes, then you must make the choice to exercise wisdom in all your health-related lifestyle habits.

OUR CHRISTIAN DUTY/PRIVILEGE

As Christians, we should be embarrassed that we are not the leaders in living exemplary, healthy lives. The Scriptures teach that, as believers, our bodies are the temple of the Holy Spirit (1 Cor. 6:19). When we are born again, the Holy Spirit comes to reside in us. As we grow in grace, we are continually filled with God for the purpose of bringing glory to Him through every area of our lives, including our physical well-being.

The apostle Paul admonishes believers to "present your bodies a living and holy sacrifice, acceptable to God, which is your spiritual service of worship" (Rom. 12:1). We understand that we are made in the likeness and image of God (Gen. 1:26). Though God does not have a physical body, His divine character should be reflected through ours by living lives that embrace His covenant promises for abundant life.

Do we as Christians embrace the Scriptures as the truth of God to be *obeyed*? Or are they convenient clichés that we use when we want to make a point, even out of context? For example, some folks are adamant about refusing to drink wine. They can quote scriptures that support their position, while helping themselves to a third doughnut that supports their unhealthy obese condition. It is not an *option* for believers to respect our body as the dwelling place of the Holy Spirit; it is an *obligation*. According to the new covenant, we are to live by this biblical principle that states clearly our lives are not our own:

> Or do you not know that your body is a temple of the Holy Spirit who is in you, whom you have from God, and that you are not your own? For you have been bought with a price: therefore glorify God in your body.
>
> —1 CORINTHIANS 6:19–20

Paul describes our physical being as the "earthen vessel" (2 Cor. 4:7) that the Lord uses to get His work done on earth. We are His arms, legs, hands, and voices to share the gospel with those who don't know Him. In short, it is the debt (and privilege) of the believer to be used as God's instrument for His purposes on earth. That is why we must position ourselves to practice wisdom in all our actions, including the area of physical health.

Why am I so passionate about this biblical truth? Physical wellness is a great way to draw attention to your newly achieved healthy lifestyle, giving you opportunity to witness for Christ. People who knew you before will applaud you when you drop fifty pounds, six dress sizes, or four notches off the belt. Coming off your blood pressure medicine, avoiding a surgery, or just not complaining about your achy back any more offer great opportunities for testimony in conversations with friends. With those opportunities comes the real impetus for your newly found attention—being able to witness to another person that both the knowledge and your motivation for applying it successfully are a result of obeying the Word of God. You can share with them the *why* of your ongoing success in maintaining a healthy lifestyle.

This reality does not in any way minimize the importance of the how-to factor of your pursuit of health. The method by which something works is critical also. I am convinced that if you follow the how-to plan presented in the later chapters of this book, the body fat will drop and the pounds will come off. You will see how the whole plan will affect your overall wellness and improve any health conditions you may have been suffering. The science behind my method is solid and makes sense from a physiological and biochemical perspective. This scientific basis is necessary to validate the effectiveness of the method.

But it is simply a fact that the science itself won't motivate would-be participants in a health protocol. The bottom line is that while science will confirm our procedures and actions, it is your correct spiritual, mental, and emotional positioning that will enhance your motivation to exercise wisdom. It is that applied knowledge that will surely bring you success. In the next chapter we will explore this concept of correct positioning that will set you free to achieve your health goals.

Chapter 2

OVERCOMING SPIRITUAL BARRIERS TO YOUR SUCCESS

I'VE INTERVIEWED THOUSANDS of patients in twenty-five years of practice, many who have come to me from other doctors. They tell me that they have tried everything and nothing seems to work. Sometimes I know the doctors they have consulted or I'm familiar with the treatment plan they were following. In those cases I am convinced that the patient's problem wasn't with the doctor or the health plan they pursued—the problem was the patient.

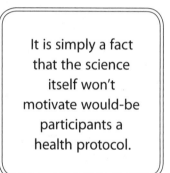

It is simply a fact that the science itself won't motivate would-be participants a health protocol.

Even if the doctor has prescribed an appropriate treatment plan, the patient may not be in the right mental or spiritual state (position) to properly follow through with the recommendations. That's why I am presenting the why factor first: to help you conquer the enemy within. Sadly, I have seen the pervasive, insidious attempts of our enemy, the devil, to destroy humanity through any means we allow. It is my intent to help you overcome any spiritual barrier to your success of which you may not even be aware.

MEDIA HYPE FAILS TO MOTIVATE TO SUCCESS

I'm sure many of you have watched those Saturday morning weight-loss infomercials on TV. I would agree that some of them are weird and have no scientific rationale for guaranteeing your success. Others are brilliant; they make me wish I had thought of marketing them first. And some infomercials make me think the marketers who created them got the idea by sneaking into my office and spying on my conversations with my patients. The truth is that a lot of these health plans will work if you *just do them*, according to the designers' recommendation.

Therein lies the problem. Most of the people *can't* successfully complete these health plans. It's not because the program doesn't work, but because the average person does not have the correct motivation to allow them to succeed. Deep-seated spiritual flaws in their lives, of which they are unaware, may weaken their motivation to pursue health. Perhaps psychologically destructive beliefs perpetually sabotage their progress. In some cases these profound spiritual and mental issues prevent people from even starting the process of getting well.

The basic formula for my health program to get into shape is relatively easy to follow successfully. Because I set it up almost as a game, it can be exciting to track your actions and measure your progress. But if you don't address these deeper issues involved in your success, when you hit bumps in the road, it may seem impossible for you to continue the plan. That is why I have designed the first several chapters of this book to help you avoid failure and to assure your success for your health goals.

In my chiropractic practice I have observed seven spiritual obstacles that can hinder your ability to be successful in reaching your health objectives. Repositioning yourself to embrace these divine principles for health is key to your correct motivation for achieving optimal health. As you consider them, I encourage you to determine whether you may be struggling with some of these issues. If you are, the good news is that becoming aware of them is the first step to conquering them. Then you will be able to reposition yourself for future success in living a life of wellness.

Spiritual Obstacle #1: Disregarding Covenant

When we read through the first five books of the Bible, called the Pentateuch, we discover a powerful attribute of God: He never changes. Among all the events and adventures of the children of Israel, God always remains a God of law and order. His rules are unwavering and exact. However, they are not strictly to execute negative judgment, but they are designed also to bless. He calls His rules for a blessed life *covenants*.

In the biblical context, a *covenant* involves promises made by God as well as divine precepts, which must be obeyed in order to enjoy the blessing of God on our lives.[1] All the covenants God establishes throughout the

Scriptures are meant to redeem mankind from sin and destruction and to give the abundant life ultimately offered through the sacrifice of Christ on Calvary for our sin. You may be familiar with what theologians refer to as the Noahic, Abrahamic, Mosaic, and Davidic covenants, among others, established between God and man in the Old Testament. In the New Testament, Jesus became the mediator of the new covenant through His blood (Heb. 12:24). He came to fulfill the law of God given to Moses and establish a better covenant. When we accept His redemption, we are free to pursue the abundant life He offers each of us.

All of God's covenant promises and precepts are given to protect us from wrong actions, wrong thinking, wrong attitudes, and negative emotional responses that have the power to bring destruction to our lives. In short, by following Christ, accepting Him as Savior, we begin to *position* ourselves to live the victorious life Christ provided for us as we submit to the Lordship of Christ. His promise of abundant life will dramatically affect our motivation toward achieving our goals for a healthy lifestyle.

In the last book of the Old Testament God declared: "For I, the LORD, do not change..." (Mal. 3:6). And the New Testament declares: "Jesus Christ is the same yesterday and today and forever" (Heb. 13:8). Just as God never changes, so His covenants with His people never change.

Throughout all the historical events and adventures of the children of Israel recorded in the Scriptures, God always remains a God of law and order. His promises and precepts are unwavering and exact. They are rules and principles for life that God gave for blessing, not for punishment. However, if they are broken, many times they carry their own consequences; in other cases we do bring the judgment of God on our disobedience.

Throughout His Word God has set up covenantal principles to direct, guide, protect, and bless the obedient soul as well as to chastise our disobedience. It is true, according to the Scriptures, that God has established His divine covenants partially to test the obedience of His people:

> And Moses said to the people, "Do not be afraid; for God has come in order to test you, and in order that the fear of Him may remain with you, so that you may not sin."
>
> —EXODUS 20:20

However, I prefer to focus on God's loving purpose through His covenantal principles to deliver on His promises of abundant life for all who do reverence Him. Our obedience to His divine principles keeps us safe and protected from the destructive purposes of the enemy. Good health is a covenantal promise of God to those who obey Him. Even those who lived under the old covenant understood their source of divine protection and physical well-being:

> And He said, "If you will give earnest heed to the voice of the Lord your God, and do what is right in His sight, and give ear to His commandments, and keep all His statutes, I will put none of the diseases on you...for I, the Lord, am your healer."
>
> —Exodus 15:26

> Fear the Lord and turn away from evil. It will be healing to your body and refreshment to your bones.
>
> —Proverbs 3:7–8

Under the new covenant, Jesus clearly declared His purpose to give to His followers abundant life:

> The thief comes only to steal and kill and destroy; I came that they might have life, and have it abundantly.
>
> —John 10:10

Sowing and reaping

You are probably familiar with the biblical analogy of sowing and reaping taught throughout the New Testament. Today we often hear the cliché: You reap what you sow. This too is a biblical principle for life:

> Do not be deceived, God is not mocked; for whatever a man sows, this he will also reap. For the one who sows to his own flesh will from the flesh reap corruption, but the one who sows to the Spirit will from the Spirit reap eternal life.
>
> —Galatians 6:7–8

This is a classic example of a covenantal principle that brings consequences or blessings. If you sow into your body acts of wellness, meaning that you eat right, exercise, and follow all the other principles that govern health, there's a good chance you will be blessed with good health. Obviously this principle works in reverse as well. If you sow destruction into your body through negative lifestyle habits, the results will be sickness and disease.

God has magnificently designed your body with such intricate detail and expertise that the most brilliant scientific minds throughout history, even to this day, still can't fully understand the basic tenets that perpetuate life. Every organ, muscle, and gland in your body has a specific function, an important task that, when working in harmony with each other, afford you optimal health. Medical science has learned 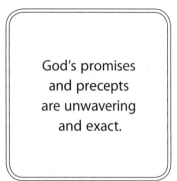 that there are things you can do to assist the proper function of your body as well as things you can do to obstruct the normal function of your body.

If you do the things you know to do that enhance the function of your body, you are being obedient to the *covenant design* that God ordained for your wellness. If you do things that are contrary to the well-being of your body, in essence you are breaking covenant with God's design for your health. Even if you do so unknowingly, you will eventually reap the consequences, which will surely result in serious dysfunction of the body. When you knowingly make conscious decisions to participate in negative lifestyle habits, you are in essence *disregarding covenant*. You may be familiar with the following classic example of how this disregard for God's covenant principles for health plays out in real life.

Everyone knows that eating ice cream every night before going to bed is not a healthy habit. And eating a few cookies along with it doesn't help. You rationalize, "But it tastes so good." You don't think it's a big deal because you wake up in the morning feeling fine. Never mind that every month you gain two or three pounds. The next day you need your two cups of coffee to get you going in the morning. You buy health supplements but forget to take them. You do have your water bottle during the day, but you need another jolt of caffeine to get you through the afternoon. That's no big deal either. "Doesn't everyone do that?"

You think about exercising but decide you're too tired from a hard and stressful day at work. "Vegging out" in front of the TV for the evening sounds like a better plan. You want to go to bed early, but your favorite show is on at 11:00 p.m., so you get to bed late, after another bowl of ice cream. When you suffer frequent back pain and headaches, instead of going to a doctor of chiropractic to correct the cause of the problem, you take pain pills. In spite of the fact they cause long-term toxicity in the body, you reason that they are convenient and less expensive than medical treatment.

In these and countless other ways, either unknowingly or intentionally, you break the covenantal laws for health that are designed to protect you from disease and allow you to live in optimal health. Sometimes, in a moment of conscience, you say to yourself, "I need to make a change." But the next day you find you are back to your old habits. The main reason people disregard the Lord's health-based covenants is that they wake up feeling OK the next day. They fail to realize the long-term damage they are inflicting on their bodies that will compound over time.

So how do you stop disregarding covenant? What will motivate you to make real changes to pursue a healthy lifestyle? As we discussed in chapter 1, you will be motivated either by *crisis* or *wisdom*—it's your choice to make!

How does this spiritual obstacle of disregarding covenantal principles specifically affect your goal of losing body fat? The challenging task of losing body fat requires a multifaceted effort, involving a willingness to change your lifestyle habits to comply with scientifically sound principles for improving your health. Your willingness to be obedient to God's covenantal principles assures the development of positive lifestyle improvement for two reasons:

1. First, developing consistent positive habits will bring consistent positive results.

2. Second, and more importantly, choosing to obey the Word of God with respect to caring for your body as the temple of the Holy Spirit will not only honor God but will also assure the success of your health goals.

OBSTACLE #2: ABUSING MERCY

Mercy, by biblical definition, means kindness, goodness, favor, pity, and compassion.[2] Mercy is a powerful, loving attribute of God that He shows to people who do not deserve it; for that reason some theologians refer to mercy as *undeserved favor*. It is rarely found in the attitudes or actions of the average man or woman. Most of us, when offended, seek retribution or revenge. In contrast, throughout the Scriptures, God is known for His great compassion in spite of mankind's continuous transgression against His Word:

> The LORD, the LORD God, compassionate and gracious, slow to anger, and abounding in lovingkindness [mercy] and truth; who keeps lovingkindness for thousands, who forgives iniquity, transgression and sin…
>
> —EXODUS 34:6–7

Of course, as a God of justice, He cannot leave the guilty unpunished (v. 7). Still, the prophet cried out to God: "…in wrath remember mercy" (Hab. 3:2). Amazingly, this concept of mercy is basic to the function of our body's divine design. The Creator of our body, who designed us in His likeness and image, built mercy into the very function of all our muscles, organs, and glands. For example, one or two nights of eating cookies and ice cream will probably not cause great physical damage; the body works hard to forgive your transgression. Some people smoke for years before the body finally succumbs to lung cancer. In these and countless ways, your body is merciful to your abuse.

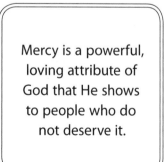

Mercy is a powerful, loving attribute of God that He shows to people who do not deserve it.

This idea of mercy built into the normal functions of our body is often, sometimes unknowingly, taken for granted. We simply expect our body to recover from the poor treatment to which we subject it. We assume that we will feel fine the next morning, as usual. Because our body is merciful regarding the ongoing abuse it receives, many people are caught in the first spiritual obstacle to optimal health we discussed, *disregarding covenant.* The sad truth is, that while the Lord's mercy may last forever, your body, or more specifically, your present good health, may not!

Every day millions of people, including Christians, have the fleeting inspiration that they are going to eat better and exercise more. They're tired of the tight-fitting clothes, the double chin, and the expanding profile they see in the mirror. They have oatmeal for breakfast, they do some sit-ups in the afternoon, and they even decide to walk home from work. But the next morning they have an early meeting, so they have no other choice but to grab a coffee and a roll; there was no time to exercise, and at the end of the day the bus was a lot more inviting than the twenty-five-minute walk home.

Can you relate to this real-life scenario? If so, you can be commended for one thing: at least you're *thinking* about the need for fitness and feebly attempting to get into shape. There are many people who don't even have the thought of improving fitness. They have no conviction at all about their poor health habits. Their philosophy fits the biblical description of people who declared, "Let us eat and drink, for tomorrow we may die" (Isa. 22:13). Except that they don't plan to die tomorrow.

People who develop a continuous habit of disregarding God's covenantal principles for health soon progress to the level of *abusing mercy.* Some people abuse their body every single day of their lives. They take for granted that their body is a self-healing mechanism and has unending resilience in spite of overwhelming physical, chemical, and emotional stress it must endure. But the physical body can only take so much. Just because the consequences of negative lifestyle habits don't show up *immediately*, it doesn't mean they are not going to catch up to you sooner or later.

What do you think researchers of heart disease do all day long? They study the correlation of poor diet and unhealthy lifestyles to the increased risk of coronary artery blockage. And you know what they find: the increased risk of heart disease for those people who are clinically obese. Therefore, not to sound like the voice of judgment, if you have been clinically obese for a while and continue to live an unhealthy lifestyle, thinking you feel OK, you may be guilty of abusing His mercy.

I know this is harsh and judgmental. There are no apologies for telling the truth. I believe you bought this book because you want to know the truth. You need to know not only how to lose a pound of body fat every three days but also how to succeed for life in achieving wellness goals. The truth is, as Christians, we should never abuse the mercy of the Lord. We should never take advantage of the wondrous healing capabilities that He has graced into our bodies.

Remember, my goal in this book is for you to get results and keep those results. I have seen thousands of people in my practice and spoken to them in my audiences who have tried everything to lose weight. They live the yo-yo life of losing weight and then gaining it back, enjoying good health and then losing it because of their return to their poor habits. The only real solution is to take personal ownership for your bad habits and develop new habits that perpetuate wellness. That's why it is imperative to be aware of the weapons the enemy wants to prosper against us (Isa. 54:17).

OBSTACLE #3: PRAYER AS A LAST RESORT

Jesus set an example of prayer that is profound, yet it is so often overlooked by believers. Throughout the Gospels there are many accounts of Jesus separating Himself from the others to go off and pray, sometimes all night. He had a great commission to fulfill, and He knew He needed to pursue extreme intimacy with God His Father. What we sometimes do not realize is that everything Jesus did was for a purpose; He lived as an example for others to follow. When we observe Jesus's priority of prayer, we learn that He always put His prayer life before His actions.

This priority of prayer seems to be missing in the life of many believers; they turn to prayer only as a last resort. Too often their actions are not based in a prayer relationship with the Lord. Much like the rest of the world, they base their actions on desires and emotions. They buy things or commit to responsibilities based on their emotional state at the moment, often regretting these decisions a few weeks later.

Others use the prayer solution as an excuse for not making a timely decision. They say, "I have to pray about it," hoping that will be accepted as a valid reason for their procrastination or outright indecision. In reality, they don't live according to Jesus's example of prayer priorities. What they really mean is, "Let me think about it to see if the decision fits comfortably into my lifestyle."

Basis for making right decisions

The fact is that some decisions you need to make, after prayerful consideration, may not be comfortable or fit smoothly into your present lifestyle. For example, assume that you come into my office for a healthy evaluation. We find that you're a perfect candidate for the Genesis Diet protocol. You acknowledge that this health plan and your present condition are a match, and you can see how you can benefit from participating in it. Next, I give you the most important information regarding the program: how long it will take and the cost. If time or money is a perceived issue, as it is with many people, you may respond that you have to go home and think about it. Or, if you are like some of my more pious patients, you may say that you have to pray about it.

After twenty-five years of practice, I have noticed that people with these considerations most often go home and try to justify why they can't follow the program recommendations. They reason, "My time and money are very precious. Is pursuing a 'non-crisis' wellness program a priority right now?" This reasoning reveals the real motivation for why they do things. While wisdom dictates that they do the program to prevent a looming health crisis, they are motivated by something other than wisdom. Unfortunately, they may soon be motivated by a previously avoidable health crisis.

I have also observed that patients who actually do pray about their decision or sincerely think about it always come back to me with a unique perspective. It is different from those who make decisions based on present circumstance or priorities. If you know in your spirit that everything about the program is right and that it would be wise to get into shape now before a crisis arises, the decision you make is always from a proactive position even if you don't feel you have the time or the money.

These patients work to overcome their circumstances in order to follow the path of wisdom. Their typical response is: "Doc, I know I need to do the program for my health and to honor the Lord, but I just don't have the money right now, and I work too late to make it happen. Is there any way I can pay you over a longer period of time to fit it into my budget? Could you make an early appointment for me before I go to work?" I suggest that we pray together for the Lord's will to give us a workable strategy to be successful. If it is the right thing to do, I am confident that the Lord will always manage a way to make it happen.

Timing of prayers

There is another aspect to overcoming this obstacle of lack of prayer; that is the timing of your prayers. Sometimes you enter into an endeavor and believe that if you just had the how-to information, that would be enough to get you to success. In later chapters you will read about the how-to of this fitness program. You will learn the science of losing weight and body fat; you will study the combination of foods to eat and the best time to eat them. And you will learn how to balance particular exercises at particular times of the day for maximum muscle performance and fat burning.

These are all part of the how-to strategy, which is simple in theory. However, completing these things requires that you overcome the stresses of your day. Your commitment to prayer for strength and guidance and for the ability to develop persistence is critical to your success before you even start the program. Your success is based on your spiritual preparation, not just the scientific method alone. You *must* put prayer first, making it a priority of life as Jesus did. Do you want to get into shape? Do you want to drop body fat? Do you want to prevent disease and premature sicknesses? Then you need to put prayer first.

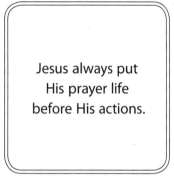

Jesus always put His prayer life before His actions.

The enemy has blinded the eyes of many Christians in this regard. They begin fitness programs to get well with halfhearted conviction, usually motivated by vanity instead of wisdom. They may achieve marginal results, then quit to look for some shortcut solution, which ultimately results in more failure. Eventually they are faced with the health crisis, the devastating diagnosis that they feared the most. As a last resort, they begin to pray. If only they would have prayed for wisdom and strength to change their lifestyle when they were still relatively healthy.

Let me exhort you, before trying the how-to strategy for wellness presented in this book, begin to make prayer your first choice, not your last resort.

OBSTACLE #4: WORKING AGAINST
CREATIVE INTELLIGENCE

I have coined the term "creative intelligence" to explain the wonderful, innate intelligence that drives the creation and development of the human body. Do you really know how your body works? I wonder if the majority of people who are non-science majors have an accurate grasp of the function and interaction of the major systems in the body. I'm not sure if all health professionals have a working knowledge of what causes disease in the body and what prevents sickness.

If you want to improve your health situation, lose some weight, lower your blood pressure naturally, or pursue freedom from other ailments, it would be a good idea to have a fundamental understanding of how the body works; it would be a sign of wisdom. However, this is often not the case. As I mentioned before, I have interviewed thousands of new patients over the years, and you would be amazed how many "well-educated" people are clueless about the basics of simple body function.

We all know that health care is a multibillion-dollar industry. Unfortunately, most of the money is spent on the treatment of diseases that could have been prevented. But is prevention really in the interest of big pharmaceutical companies and giant hospital conglomerates? Of course not. So billions of dollars are pumped into the media with a single purpose: sell the medicine or sell the procedure.

Every day you watch dozens of commercials that promote drugs for asthma, allergies, headaches, sinus trouble, high cholesterol, acid reflux, constipation, back pain, depression, and scores of other ailments. Never will they suggest that you seek out a safer, more natural alternative before you purchase their product. Never will they suggest that you attempt to determine the *cause* of the ailment and then make natural lifestyle changes before you fill a prescription to treat the *symptoms*. Even when, by law, they mention the potential side effects, they make it sound like the consumer really shouldn't worry.

When I see these ads, all I can say is, "Are you kidding me?" The side effects are often more serious than the condition. Are you telling me that taking an asthma drug that can cause a stroke or blood clot is not a serious risk? I personally would rather have a wheeze in my chest than a blood clot in my brain. Maybe the person should change their diet first and add some natural supplements that will remove the neurological interference in the spine affecting the lungs and adrenal glands. These treatments are all safe, natural, and scientifically sound. Most importantly, they have no dangerous side effects.

The innate healing power of the body

The real problem of epidemic health issues is a lack of knowledge or a loss of knowledge. Thousands of commercials, magazine ads, and TV programs are brainwashing the population with their pharmaceutical propaganda. They deny that the Creator who made the body can heal the body with its innate, built-in healing mechanisms. They insist that a drug, pill, or potion must be administered to the body to cover up the symptoms or alter the function of organs, glands, and systems.

The truth is that the human body, by its very design, is a self-sustaining, self-healing mechanism. Our Creator constructed the brain as the master control system that instructs and coordinates every function of every muscle, organ, and gland in the body. The cardiovascular system, the respiratory system, and the immune system are made up of a variety of organs and glands. They operate in a complicated but synchronized fashion, perfectly coordinated to achieve normal function and optimal health. All the actions and coordination of hormones and other chemicals are explicitly managed by neurological signals generated from the brain. It sounds intense and complicated, and in reality, it is much more complicated than I just summarized. The greatest scientific research minds on earth are continuously amazed at the sophisticated function and untapped power of the human brain.

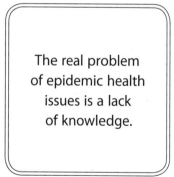

The real problem of epidemic health issues is a lack of knowledge.

In the very beginning of embryonic development, the primitively formed brain and spinal cord start the process of coordinating the development of the embryo into a fetus. Stem cells, by some yet-to-be-understood mechanism that I like to call *God's creative intelligence*, cause these cells to change and form more specific cells, eventually to be recognized as building blocks for various muscles, organs, and glands. In the end, the body's innate creative intelligence, stored and generated from the neurological system, controls the exact development or creation of your entire body.

Now it just makes sense that if a power or intelligence created your body from two cells (the sperm and the egg), this intelligence can direct healing throughout the body as long as there is no neurological or chemical interference. So, if you want to achieve optimal wellness, it follows that you must work *with* your creative intelligence, not against it.

Because God Himself designed your body's creative intelligence, it is in complete compliance with His divine covenant and all the principles that govern wellness. Disregarding covenant to adopt detrimental lifestyle habits all work against your body's innate creative intelligence and results in interference capable of developing disease. For example, taking medications without correcting lifestyle habits will only lead to further dysfunction in the body.

I understand that in some cases the level of neglect or injury has caused enough "limitation of matter" that even if you correct all your lifestyle habits, the damage may be irreversible, apart from God's divine intervention. For example, in the case of diabetes that has led to arterial damage, causing blindness or requiring amputation, there is no way to retrieve this loss of matter apart from a creative miracle. Perhaps a patient has only one kidney or has had a lung removed, suffered a stroke or paralysis due to a bullet wound. In that case, medication is necessary to maintain function and in some cases life itself.

Still, optimal wellness is achieved when you work *with* the creative intelligence of the body, not against it. In the case of improving your metabolism, for example, there are some basic parameters governed by science to which you must adhere. If you increase your intake of calories so that they are greater than the amount you burn, you will probably gain weight; if you consume less calories than you burn, you will probably lose weight. It is important to realize that whatever you do to improve your health, you need to make sure you are working with your body's creative intelligence and not against it.

From now on, every time you go to the doctor, I suggest you ask him or her two candid questions: "Doctor, do you know the cause of my problem?" And, "Is the treatment you're recommending designed to correct the cause or simply to treat the symptoms?" Regardless of the answer, at least you know where you stand and can be better prepared to make health decisions.

OBSTACLE #5: BELIEVING EVERYTHING YOU HEAR

Most of us make decisions based on our accumulated knowledge or our trust in someone we believe has the knowledge to make correct decisions. This is seen classically in the world of health care decisions. People will make decisions regarding their health based on information they learned in school, experienced in past encounters with health conditions, and through what they have heard for years from media bombardment. Of course, they may also take the advice of doctors they trust.

We must be careful that the things we believe, which form the basis for our decisions, don't contradict our ability to exercise faith in God when it comes to receiving divine healing. Just a few paragraphs ago we discussed the power of the creative intelligence that is innate to our bodies, with its incredible ability to restore and regenerate health. The very development of our physical body, from conception to birth, is a testimony to the amazing power of this creative intelligence in the body. In today's medical world, there has been this massive turn to dependency on man-made medications for every ailment imaginable. Have you ever wondered how in the world humanity made it this far with out all these prescription drugs? I am not anti-pharmaceutical. I am simply pointing out that our culture has become one of anti-trust in the body's innate ability to heal itself. It is more important than ever that you don't believe everything you hear, even if you hear it a thousand times.

Everywhere you turn there is an overload of the "treat the symptoms" message from TV commercials, radio spots, newspaper ads, and magazine articles. Then we have the "hero doctor" shows where lives are saved in bustling emergency rooms and cavalier diagnosticians cure mysterious diseases. This all makes for good TV, and I am grateful that in some cases the good results portrayed in these programs are actually true.

However, the downside is that there's a different reality being set up in the mind of the viewer. The average person is getting flooded with a subliminal message that actually diminishes their ability to exercise faith in God's healing power or trust the body's innate ability to heal itself. Like it or not, the underlying message of the health culture today is, "There is nothing you can do to help yourself get well. That is why you need our product." Here are some examples of their claims:

- Diet and exercise are not enough; you need our product to lower your cholesterol.

- When you can't get to sleep, you need our pills to get a good night's sleep.

- The pollen is making you sneeze; our pills can stop the symptoms.

- You're feeling depressed and having mood swings; don't worry, our pills will make you happy.

- Can't perform like you use to? Our pill will make you a teen-ager again.

- Can't lose weight? It's not your fault. Our pill will curb your appetite, speed up your metabolism, and build lean muscles without exercise.

Thousands of times a week pharmaceutical and medical vendors tell you: "You need our pill, potion, or surgical procedure in order to feel or look better." This is marketing at its finest. The goal is to get you to buy their products, primarily. They are not overtly trying to sabotage your faith in God. But many times that is exactly what happens. Over time this philosophical message of receiving health from a pill will eventually sink in and be accepted as the ultimate truth.

Why should you work so hard on getting into shape and maintaining good health? If your blood pressure gets a little high, there's a drug that will fix that; if the headache persists, well, there's a drug for that also. This is becoming more and more the universal thought process, regardless of your personal faith tradition. As a Christian, you need to be on guard and establish a correct set of beliefs when making decisions regarding your health.

Respect your body as the temple of God.

First, you should truly respect your body as the temple of the Holy Spirit (1 Cor. 6:19). That means you must determine to change your lifestyle habits so they line up with the covenantal principles that govern good health. That includes eating better, exercising, learning to avoid toxins, and practicing good principles for your overall health.

Secondly, if you do get sick, you must believe that God is still in the healing business. So, whatever health care program you choose, you must focus on removing the *cause* of your ailment first and then treating the symptoms. This is a critical point, because if you just treat your symptoms and allow the cause of your problem to slowly get worse over time, eventually what might have been a preventable condition will become an irreversible disease. This focus, in reality, is a spiritual position that must be enforced. Honor God in your body by doing what is right on a daily basis.

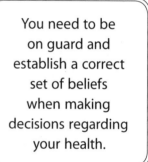

You need to be on guard and establish a correct set of beliefs when making decisions regarding your health.

What you believe determines your success.

You may be saying to yourself, "Why is Dr. V going through all this hoopla on spiritual principles just to teach me to lose body fat? Why doesn't he just cut to the chase and show me how to do it?" The reason is, *I want you to be successful.* What I have seen in my experience is that patients who do not recognize and address these spiritual obstacles or patients with a failure-based mentality (intentionally or unintentionally) never achieve lasting results. On the other hand, patients who become aware of these spiritual pitfalls and adjust their mental disposition to a success-based perspective always get great and lasting results. So you be the judge. Is it more important to just provide good health information that you will never use? Or give you a success formula that will help you achieve anything you attempt? It is simply a fact that what you believe (the "why" factor) determines your success.

Sadly, there is little evidence that Christians overall are any healthier, take fewer medications, or live longer and enjoy a better quality of life than the rest of the population. Even non-Christians who live a covenant-based healthy lifestyle will inevitably be healthier than people who don't.

My desire is for believers to wake up and realize that God has set before them a comprehensive plan that involves changing their mind-set, spiritual position, and mental outlook to receive the covenant blessings of His Word for health. Submitting to these simple truths of God has the ability to maximize health.

The Genesis Diet, as a method of losing body fat, is just a stepping-stone to realizing the divine health God has ordained for you. God has wonderfully made your body for His good pleasure so you can accomplish the good work He planned in your life and bring glory to Him in all you do. For you to succeed in God's plan for you, it is imperative that you choose to believe His Word and not to believe everything else you hear.

SPIRITUAL OBSTACLE #6: HARBORING THE ENEMY

Now this sounds harsh! During wartime, harboring the enemy is considered an act of treason. You are expected to give no place of safety to the enemy; if you do, you have betrayed your country. As an analogy to the health of your body, harboring the enemy is not a formula for success. In reality, harboring the enemy is a strategy that will result in death.

The enemies you may be harboring, consciously or unconsciously, that threaten your health are negative emotions; deep-seated emotions in your soul profoundly affect your attitudes, actions, and decisions. These negative emotions do not resemble the fruit of the Holy Spirit: love, joy, peace, patience, kindness, goodness, faithfulness, gentleness, self-control (Gal. 5:22–23). Rather, they are a result of the relentless work of the adversary against your soul to get you to harbor the enemies of resentment, bitterness, and unforgiveness that are scientifically proven to be a detriment to your health.

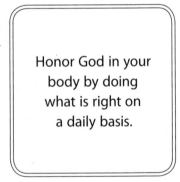

Honor God in your body by doing what is right on a daily basis.

The enemy wants you to give in to harboring anger, guilt, fear, jealousy, envy, and other negative emotions and destructive attitudes that will dictate the way you think and act. Destructive attitudes that fuel low self-esteem and hopelessness are a perfect recipe for failure.

You are probably aware how these attitudes and emotions can sabotage relationships and threaten promotion in your vocation or employment. But how often do you consider how harboring these powerful enemies can be self-destructive to your physical body? People who hold on to these emotions and attitudes only hurt themselves. Their manifestation, resulting in profoundly destructive health habits, is a reality that I see in patients every day.

Consequences of harboring the enemy

If you're not in great shape and you want to get into great shape, you need to make some physical changes. But more importantly, you will need to make some mental, emotional, spiritual, and attitudinal transformations. In the process of losing weight, dropping body fat, and improving your fitness, you will experience stresses and feel opposition against your success. Problems on your job, stresses in the family, and just everyday conflicts are always looming to test your patience and resolve. If you're harboring enemy-fueled emotions, feelings, and attitudes, there's a good chance they will have the power to break even your strongest resolve to pursue a healthy lifestyle.

I see this in my practice. Patients come in who are gung ho on getting into shape. They're doing all the right things, acting according to plan, and even dropping serious weight faster than they thought possible. Then all of a sudden, the weight stops dropping, their fervor is dampened, and their resolve to continue is shaken. Something has happened to threaten their initial steadfast disposition toward improving their health. Maybe someone in his or her family offended them and broke their trust again. Hurt feelings and negative emotions arise and consume their thoughts. Their ability to concentrate is rattled. And they give in to a "What's the use?" attitude.

As emotional beings, we often act and make decisions based entirely on our emotional reactions. Unfortunately, what happens quite often is that a negative emotional reaction to one aspect of your life produces a destructive reaction in an entirely unrelated aspect of your life. Granted, if you are hurt or offended, it is natural to be angry. It may take awhile to process the hurt and choose to forgive the offense. But if you choose to harbor that offense and refuse to release it to the Lord, your negative response will only hurt you in the long run.

For example, often I see in patients such powerful whelming up of the negative emotion that it can change their proposed menu from salad to pizza, their exercise plan from an hour on the treadmill to two hours watching TV. Then malaise sets in, and people become ambivalent about their commitment to getting into shape. I have found that, while people react with different negative emotions or attitudes, taken together, these are the most common disrupters of any wellness or fitness program. Negative emotional reactions nearly always manifest in some type of destructive behavior directed either against one's self or against another person.

The key to overcoming this barrier to your success is to become critically aware of this common phenomenon and then follow these two steps:

1. First, you must separate the negative emotion (not an attribute of God) from your actions, especially those involving health habits.

2. Second, if you are aware that the negative emotion is not going away, it may be time for a Holy Spirit intervention. You may need the assistance of a mature Christian leader to counsel and pray with you.

The important point is to never harbor these enemies; don't allow a negative emotion to fester in your spirit. The enemy may trick you into believing that these negative responses give you power against your enemy. It is a false sense of power that blinds you to the true enemy; i.e., the negative emotion and attitude you are harboring within you. They are a bomb ticking away in your soul that will lead eventually to your own destruction.

Again, my goal is to have you succeed in the how-to-live-in-optimal-health by understanding the why. Many people try to turn their health around with diets, exercise, and other means, but much too often they fall terribly short of their goals. Only 3 to 5 percent of those who try commercial weight-loss or fitness programs actually achieve lasting results over a five-year period of time. Of the 95 percent who fail, many keep trying new approaches, hoping they find the magic easy-to-do formula to a trimmer waistline. In the end, the problem is not the *program*

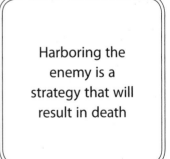

Harboring the enemy is a strategy that will result in death

but how the person is *programmed*. Harboring the enemies of negative emotions and attitudes program them for failure, which could ultimately lead to their untimely death.

Spiritual Obstacle #7: Speaking Death

It is important to realize the Word of God, His written covenant, which is truth, is in action even if you don't know that covenant or understand it. Jesus said that when you know the truth, it will set you free (John 8:32). The Word of God is "living and active and sharper than any two-edged sword, and piercing as far as the division of soul and spirit, of both joints and marrow, and able to judge the thoughts and intentions of the heart" (Heb. 4:12). It will set you free from speaking death as you allow it to judge your thoughts and intentions.

Scripture teaches clearly that "death and life are in the power of the tongue, and those who love it will eat its fruit" (Prov. 18:21). In essence this means that there is such power in the words that we choose to say that they have the ability to create life or produce death.

Speaking death is the easiest obstacle to detect, but it is one of the toughest to correct. Whenever I interview a patient, it doesn't take very long for me to realize whether this patient is one who speaks life or one who speaks death. One of the simple telltale phrases is "I can't." Other variations are "I don't have" or "I am" (followed by "a diabetic" or other disease from which they suffer). Then there is the infamous failure-prone phrase "I'll try." Whenever I hear these and similar expressions, I immediately turn to my whiteboard and boldly write the words, DON'T SPEAK DEATH. Then I turn back to the patient without saying a word. This response usually gets their attention. The next thing I often hear is, "What do you mean, 'Don't speak death'?"

Kindly I explain, "Whatever you believe and is fixed in your heart is what brews into your mind and eventually comes out of your mouth. Jesus said in Matthew 12:34, 'The mouth speaks out of that which fills the heart.' The spoken word becomes the affirmation of what you think you can't or won't be able to do."

If you want to lose weight, get into shape, and prevent or reverse disease, you must first eliminate certain confessions from your vernacular. This does not mean you ignore a brain tumor or the symptoms of a heart attack.

What I mean is, you must stop reinforcing the negative and be mindful of speaking life. For example, in approaching your health plan, begin to speak positive affirmations of your pending success, your resolve to reach your goals, and other thoughts of life, which will create hope in your heart. Be careful to avoid saying:

- "I can't do..." because you don't have the ability right now.

- "I don't have..." because you lack the resources right now.

- "I am diabetic or I have heart disease," defining your life in this negative way.

Instead, begin to work on saying, "I am challenged with finding a solution for handling my sugar problem and a possible malfunction with my pancreas, but I am continuing to seek a solution." Or, "I am working to minimize or reverse the onset of heart disease by getting into shape." Speaking positive goals is good practice to motivate the subconscious mind to seek solutions and modify destructive behavior.

Awareness is imperative to your success.

It is sad to me that many people fail to reach their health goals and do not understand why. This lack of understanding compounds their frustration and leads to more failure. It is imperative that you be mindful of these seven spiritual obstacles to your success. Much too often we try to go right for the "meat and potatoes" (which is a bad choice of words for a book that promotes wellness) and learn the how-to as fast as possible to get results. If that were a correct formula, there wouldn't be a new weight-loss product needed; those on the market now would have succeeded for everyone who tried them.

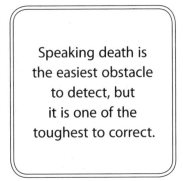

Speaking death is the easiest obstacle to detect, but it is one of the toughest to correct.

The reason most plans, potions, and programs can't deliver what you expect is that they don't deliver to you what you *should* expect. The producers of most wellness programs try to sell you on the breakthrough science and the high-speed results. They fail to mention the pitfalls, obstacles, and hazards that could hinder your success. Patients who have tried these programs too often end up in my office seeking answers to their failure. My focus is on your long-term success, not a flash-in-the-pan loss of ten pounds jump-start program that proves to be unsustainable. Spiritual preparation and positioning are integral to the success of your health plan, as well as biblical principles for its implementation and successful completion, which we will discuss in the next chapter.

Chapter 3

YOUR "GET INTO SHAPE" SUCCESS ATTITUDES

HOPEFULLY, YOU WERE able to navigate through chapter 2 with an open mind and willing spirit, determined to overcome any of the spiritual obstacles you identified to your success. It's not always easy to be completely transparent and honest with yourself. But in order to reach your optimal health goals, you must conquer the why factors that would defeat you otherwise.

In the last chapter we showed you the importance of overcoming spiritual obstacles to your success in achieving wellness goals, and in life. In this chapter, we're going to discuss eight essential principles that you need to cultivate, which are essential for achieving your goals of living the abundant life. These covenantal principles, which form the basis for what I call your *success attitude*, are taken from powerful lessons Abraham learned in his obedience to God's difficult assignment.

You may be familiar with the account of Abraham's son of promise (covenant) that God miraculously gave to him and Sarah, his wife, after they were much too old to become parents. In spite of all the promises God gave to Abraham regarding Isaac, who was to become Abraham's heir, one day God told Abraham to take his beloved son to a mountain and sacrifice him there. Abraham simply obeyed God's command. But when he raised the knife to kill the son he loved, God spoke to him not to do it. He had been testing Abraham's obedience and his character and now knew that Abraham feared God. God Himself provided a ram for the sacrifice he had required of Abraham. (See Genesis 22:1–14.)

The following eight principles, drawn from this account of Abraham's obedience in the face of a supremely difficult choice, are necessary for success in any pursuit in life. I am convinced that if you abide by these principles with steadfast integrity, you will be successful in completing the Genesis Diet, as well as anything else you attempt in your life. After discussing these eight success attitudes, I will summarize them in light of Abraham's awesome experience.

SUCCESS ATTITUDE #1: NO MORE EXCUSES

The attitude of "no more excuses" is one of the most important attitudes to have in order to reach your goals. Almost everyone who needs to lose weight also has the desire to lose weight. But many of them have convinced themselves of a legitimate excuse for why they can't get started on a weight-loss program. Then, many who do get past the inertia of not starting quit soon after at the first signs of stress.

This habit of making excuses, which is directly related to Spiritual Obstacle #7: Speaking Death, has several extenuating circumstances. First, if the excuse is based on laziness or a desire not to be inconvenienced, it plays into the pitfall of speaking negative thoughts of doom. Next, many excuses are simply justifications for poor management of priorities. And finally, if you speak the excuse enough times, you may actually start believing your own delusion.

So how does making excuses affect your resolve of getting into shape? Achieving health goals can mean many things to different people. For one person, it can mean a nonchalant, low-priority goal of losing five or ten pounds. Nothing seems urgent to them, and there are no big or immediate consequences for not following through. For another person, getting into shape is a matter of life or death; they have no options. And many others find themselves somewhere on this spectrum from low to high priority of pursuing health goals. They may exercise two of the most common excuses for not getting into shape, the degree or intensity of those excuses being determined by this priority of their health goals.

"I don't have the money."

The first common excuse is, "I don't have the money." The person reasons that the amount of money he is asked to spend is greater than the perceived gain (reward) at the present time. If getting into shape is a low-priority matter, than spending high-priority money is not a match. The problem with this value system is that it follows the faulty reasoning, "If I'm not in crisis mode, what's the urgency of spending the money?"

Promoting your good health is an investment into your future. That doesn't mean you have to spend a fortune on a treadmill; you can walk around the track at the local high school. However, the sad fact is that being stingy when it comes to your health will always, always come back to haunt you. One of the biggest mistakes I hear patients make is saying, "Maybe it will go away," not understanding that it cannot go away unless they choose to correct the cause of a problem.

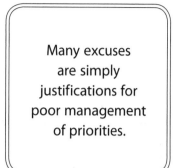

Many excuses are simply justifications for poor management of priorities.

The *symptoms* may go away for a while, but the cause usually gets worse if not addressed appropriately. In the end, the problem can become ten times worse and cost a hundred times more for treatment, if it is still treatable. It is prudent to use wisdom. Evaluate all the things you need to do or that need to get done. Take a good look at where your health is on your list of priorities and see if it needs to move up a notch.

"I don't have the time."

The second common excuse is, "I don't have the time." Some may consider this their first excuse, but experience teaches that spending of money usually directs the spending of time. However, our spending of time is also allocated to activities and actions based on their perceived level of priority. Much too often, time is assigned to actions that give the greatest amount of pleasure in the shortest period of time with the least amount of effort. As a matter of fact, this concept is also often consistent with how we spend our money as well.

Again, a crisis-motivated person, who at the present time is asymptomatic, would never spend two thousand dollars on an intense eight-month wellness course. That's too much money to spend and too much time involvement. Where do we find that person three years later who didn't change their diet, never did any exercise, and just lived life with an "if it ain't broke, don't fix it" attitude? One day they're dizzy, nauseated, and can't catch their breath. They go to the emergency room, and after eight hours, six diagnostic tests, and seven thousand dollars in medical fees, their diagnosis is acute diabetic shock.

What an overall shock! The moral of the story is to remember that good health is an investment in your future requiring both time and money. Spending a little money now will save you a fortune in medical bills later. And spending a little consistent time now will add plenty of healthy years to your life.

SUCCESS ATTITUDE #2: TAKE INITIATIVE NOW

When God told Abraham to take Isaac to the mountain and prepare a sacrifice, he packed the boy up and left. The biblical account says, "So Abraham rose early in the morning…and went to the place of which God had told him" (Gen. 22:3). Without making excuses, Abraham just got up and went to fulfill a most difficult assignment. In that same way, when the Father told Jesus, His Son, that it was time to go to Jerusalem to be crucified, Jesus went. He knew this was the beginning of the end. He knew it was His last week. There was no discussion or excuse making, just simple, immediate obedience to the Father's will. Abraham and Jesus exemplified the principle of highest obedience in their immediate response to fulfill the most difficult of divine assignments.

Have you ever heard the adage "There's no time like the present"? The truth is, the best time for you to get into shape is NOW. Occasionally I have a few people come up to me after a conference and give me the "great conference, Doc, love to join the program, but I think I'll start maybe next month" story. My response is often, "There's no time like the present." This answer, of course, usually sparks the antithesis of Success Attitude #1, a barrage of almost believable excuses.

Let me clarify that there are some legitimate reasons for not starting a "get healthy now" program. But if they relate to no time or no money, they are usually excuses based on a lack of priority and sense of urgency. The problem with not taking immediate initiative is the ever-looming spirit of procrastination that stalks you. You have probably heard the maxim, "Don't put off for tomorrow what can be done today." This is the ideal quote for people who think that tomorrow is a better time to start getting into shape. Tomorrow turns into a week, a week into a year, and a year turns into, "Oh my God, I have the disease I thought I would never get."

The time to take care of your health is NOW. The day to start eating better and exercising is TODAY. Never let another tomorrow rob today. Do any of us know our last day, week, or year? Can you determine that you still have six months before enough plaque builds up in your arteries that it is still reversible? Taking initiative to improve your health *now* is the wisdom that prevents the impending crisis. Do not create a regretful memory of "I should have" or "If only I would have listened."

SUCCESS ATTITUDE #3: WILLINGNESS TO MAKE SACRIFICES

This success attitude can meet with some strong innate resistance because it directly bucks against our human nature to satisfy self. It is part of our nature to want to be drawn toward pleasure and to move away from pain. This is most obviously seen when we are faced with an immediate or short-term decision promising instant self-gratification.

For example, when faced with a decision to eat because we feel hungry at the same time that we are stressed, our decision would naturally be to instantly satisfy both matters at hand. Fill the stomach and uplift the emotions. This usually translates into eating a lot of the wrong kind of food that is very tasty and usually fattening.

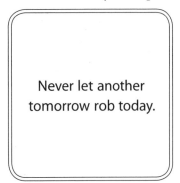

Never let another tomorrow rob today.

Your willingness to make sacrifices is a key principle to your success in all of life—especially regarding your health. This success attitude impacts significantly the seven spiritual obstacles we discussed in chapter 2. If you are struggling with one or more of those spiritual obstacles, where your faith is being challenged, you need to determine to win this spiritual battle. Otherwise it will be difficult for you to make sacrifices for your health. If your perception of how your body works is ill-informed or if you have been in the habit of speaking negative statements and sabotaging your own faith, you may also find it very difficult to make conscious sacrifices.

In these situations it is imperative that you be honest and transparent with yourself. For example, you're faced with a decision to take a positive step, like eating a piece of fruit instead of a handful of cookies. But you choose the unhealthy action instead, wolfing down the cookies. Don't give in to an attitude of regret or remorse; begin to identify your *internal motivating factor* that swayed your decision to eat the cookies instead of the fruit. Why were the cookies going to give you more satisfaction or pleasure than the healthier fruit?

When you begin to think in terms of your motivation, you will find that most of the time there is an emotional issue that you associate with pain or displeasure lurking underneath your decision. You think that the taste of the cookies somehow has the ability to counterbalance that feeling of displeasure. Some people call it "eating comfort foods."

> Your willingness to make sacrifices is a key principle to your success in all of life.

How do you win this battle against wrong *internal* motivating factors? Well, forget about just trying to resist them in your own willpower. Instead, work to create or discover powerful *external* motivating factors. These factors usually take the form of short-term goals, which require tasks that are not pleasurable—sacrifices—that will result in long-term success and pleasure. They can also be a strong personality trait that helps to motivate you to achieve your goals, which I will discuss later. Let me explain.

Short-term goals

Consider this hypothetical scenario. You get an e-mail invitation to your twenty-fifth high school reunion, scheduled in three months. The person who sent the e-mail was a very popular, although irritating, classmate who just happened to include a recent personal photo on a beach in Maui. You can't get the picture of that forty-two-year-old classmate with the twenty-two-year-old body out of your head. This image becomes an excellent *external motivating factor* to make you willing to make sacrifices. It creates a short-term goal to avoid being "shown up" at the reunion.

Of course, you can decline the invitation and follow your *internal* motivating factor to instant gratification, eating another slice of pizza. You could also Google the easiest crash diet you can find that promises unrealistic results with potential for damaging your long-term health. Or you can use this goal as a very powerful driving force to make the short-term sacrifices necessary to get into the best shape you can in the next three months—and forever.

Real life-changing success often occurs when you are able to string multiple external motivating factors together (either real or self-fabricated), choosing to intentionally place yourself into a situation of accountability to achieve your long-term health goals. The pain of your short-term sacrifices to eat better, exercise, and become more health conscious overall is soon forgotten in your newfound pleasure of looking and feeling great. Remember, it is God's desire that you succeed in your goals to live His abundant life.

It is important to realize that you are in a fight, a battle. You need to believe that you are not a slave to your negative emotions, which demand you indulge in unhealthy eating habits to achieve immediate satisfaction. Then you need to prepare for the battle to make a sacrifice by finding your external motivating factor and creating a strategy around it to be successful. Intentional preparation helps you avoid the stress caused by making tough decisions; your determined choices ease the pain of the sacrifice.

Strong personality traits

I mentioned that your external motivating factor may be a strong personality trait that can stimulate a positive reaction; it can be a powerful enough motivating force to subdue even a long-standing negative habit. Establishing a new positive habit in its place will eventually eliminate the perception of sacrifice. Here is an example.

I have a patient named Big Ray who vehemently hated to exercise. He would make every excuse in the book for why he couldn't, shouldn't, and wouldn't exercise. He was the poster boy for the sedentary lifestyle. The challenge was to discover what external motivating factor could push him to exercise. As I got to know Ray, I found out that he had been a college basketball star. For many years he had coached high school basketball. I discovered Ray had been a very competitive player and coach; he didn't like to lose. But that competitive trait had not translated into the area of his health goals; he had chosen a lifestyle that was making him lose his health little by little.

When I learned about Ray's competitiveness (external motivating factor), I challenged him to a game of basketball. I told him that I was going to kill him, that he wouldn't even score a point. Now Ray was not going to allow his "trash-talking doctor" to get the best of him. Ray is eighteen years my senior, but he is six feet eight inches and wasn't going to stand for me to get the best of him. Ray's competitive personality kicked in, and he began to exercise every day, not for improving his health, but so that he could compete with me on the basketball court.

In addition, I reinforced this external motivating factor every week when he came into my office for care. I would always make some teasing remark about our someday challenge. Ray, the man who hated to exercise, was now spending twenty-five minutes twice a week exercising in the gym at my office.

Before my challenge, it was a huge sacrifice to get Ray off the couch to do even three minutes of simple exercises. But once we discovered his competitive nature, he was a different man. Doing exercise was no longer a great sacrifice; it became a necessary task to achieve a necessary goal—to beat his doctor on the basketball court.

In summary, to develop this success attitude, you need to:

1. Determine that this is a battle and that you are prepared to fight.

2. Identify negative *internal motivating factors.*

3. Find or create a powerful *external motivating factor.*

4. Establish a strategy for health that satisfies your external motivating factor.

Your chances of success are always increased when you have someone to support you through the process and when you make yourself accountable. (See Success Attitude #8.) You can take a moment to go to our website at www.schoolofwellness.com and watch the brief video about the Genesis Diet online support program. We are there to help you. And never forget that the Lord wants you to succeed because He has a vested interest in your well-being. Your body is His temple!

SUCCESS ATTITUDE #4: NO MORE SHORTCUTS

Slow incremental changes based on wisdom are the only sound and lasting solution to your health problems. You will see this principle reiterated throughout this text. It is the only effective method for lifelong success. The world around us is constantly trying to persuade us that there is a shortcut to losing weight and gaining health. People have been trained by the media hype to hope that soon there will be an easier, quicker, and less expensive way to get rapid results. The truth is, their promised shortcuts rarely, if ever, work for long-term success. The end result is usually failure and disappointment.

If you've ever turned on your TV on Saturday morning, you will notice that many channels are airing infomercials. Many of these programs are focusing on health, primarily weight loss and beauty. The goal of these infomercials is to persuade the audience that they have discovered a "breakthrough" or "revolutionary" product or service that will be able to give you, the potential customer, unbelievable quick results.

> Slow incremental changes based on wisdom are the only sound and lasting solution to your health problems.

Their main goal is to convince you that your two main excuses (no time, no money) are invalid. They tell you that you can get their breakthrough product, valued at five hundred dollars for only fifty dollars if you act now; it only takes five minutes a day to complete, and other equally outrageous claims. I have observed six critical aspects to these infomercials that you should consider.

CRITICAL ASPECTS OF BREAKTHROUGH INFOMERCIAL CLAIMS

- The "you're not going to believe it, but it's true" claim
- The dozens of testimonies of how simple and easy it was to do; if they can do it, anyone can.
- The "it's not expensive," "it doesn't take a lot of effort," "it replaces everything else," "it won't disrupt your lifestyle," "you can still eat whatever you want," "it only takes a few minutes per day," and "you need to act now because this offer won't last!" hype.

- The "if you're not completely satisfied, you can get your money back, but keep the free gift" promise

- The small print, barely legible disclaimer that shows up in the background that reads, "These are not typical results."

- "I did it like they said, and I am so disappointed."

The sixth critical aspect to the infomercial claims is perhaps the most devastating: the disappointment! I'm not saying that every advertised diet, exercise machine, workout DVD, super supplement, or packaged meal is a waste and a fraud. What I'm saying is that the marketing of the product or service is very deceptive. They focus on addressing the most common excuses for why people don't get into shape: no time, no money. Then they play on negative human emotions and personality traits. Most people love to get a great deal—instant gratification, something for nothing, hit the lottery, and "Where's my free lunch?" It has been ingrained in our very fiber to be on the lookout for every shortcut life has to offer. Be honest and tell me if you can relate to the following:

1. Everyone is so busy and we have no time to do anything. So why go to the gym and spend hours every day for months when with the "Super ABC Exerciser" and twenty-minutes-a-day workout, I'll have six-pack abs in eight weeks just like the person in the testimonial.

2. Everyone loves to save money and get a great bargain. The "Super Macho Workout DVDs" look awesome, and what a great price. To join the gym will cost hundreds of dollars per year, and to get a trainer to personally show me what I can do on the video would cost me thousands. The DVD package is only "three easy payments of $39.95," and "that's not all." You also get the two bonus DVDs, the menu planner, and the Super Macho exercise rubber band.

3. No one likes to break an unnecessary sweat. Why work out all day if I can just use the "breakthrough device" for one-fourth the time? Why shop and cook when I can just order the meals online? Why eat so-called "healthy foods" when I can just take the "breakthrough supplement" instead?

4. No one likes to step out of his or her comfort zone. The thought of seeing a change in your weight, increasing muscle mass, experiencing better-moving bowels, and enjoying healthier skin without making any change to your daily routine is quite an enticing promise.

The idea of the shortcut, or more specifically the selling of the shortcut, is presented from a work-less, pay-less, stress-less, do-less, and sweat-less perspective. The exercise devices, DVDs, and the weight-loss programs that are promoted in the shortcut may in themselves be great products and services. But the perception advertisers project is that you can behave in a mediocre fashion and still get great results.

This projection, of course, is farthest from the truth. That's why they have to include the disclaimer about "not typical results." Even though they market their products to the mediocre, underachiever mind-set, the people who give the testimonials are not representative of that mind-set. They are more than likely highly motivated overachievers who were fed up with their situation. An analysis of their personalities would most likely reveal, consciously or unconsciously, that they have succeeded in avoiding the spiritual obstacles discussed in chapter 2 and most definitely operated in all the success attitudes we are discussing in this chapter.

Some people learn these principles for success simply by reading and applying them (deriving wisdom from other people), and some learn experientially (deriving wisdom from the their own experiences). Please understand that I'm not a total fan of the idea that hard work always pays off. I'm more a fan of the idea that *smart* hard work always pays off. And smart hard work means following the principles and attitudes that we are discussing that assure long-term success, achieving your health goals, and living the abundant life Jesus promised.

Success Attitude #5: Stick to the Plan—and Own It

If the plan makes sense both scientifically and emotionally, you must be willing to stick to the plan to be successful. Changing the plan to make it more *convenient* usually does not lead to success. This is the mistake that many people make. They are initially convinced that the plan of action they are going to take to get into shape is perfect. It addresses all the issues of exercise, diet, and other procedures and treatments, which have been proven to work. But after the first week of their participation, they realize that the plan or program they're doing is interfering with their daily routine. Or they discover that some of the preparatory steps they need to take actually require more time than they expected.

At this point they are tempted to adjust the program to their lifestyle. When this happens, it is time to STOP and review the purpose behind the plan. They need to consider the covenant principles and success attitudes presented here. Otherwise, excuses will begin to pop up, and their ability to make sacrifices will become compromised. They will be looking for shortcuts or personal changes to make the plan more convenient and less stressful.

Making personal adjustments to a proven plan is not always a bad idea if the changes you make are not compromising to the plan and not just done out of convenience. Over the past ten years I have painstakingly worked on developing a comprehensive, detailed program for my patients to get into shape. It has proven to be successful for

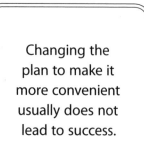

Changing the plan to make it more convenient usually does not lead to success.

many of them. Still, there are some aspects of the plan that are flexible and may be altered due to personal preference. There are also aspects that are written in stone and cannot be changed to achieve the success desired.

Doing it right

Denise started off my program like a champ. The first two weeks she ate the exact foods used as examples in the sample food chart. I thought that was kind of bizarre, because the purpose of the chart is simply to show you how to record the foods you eat; it was not meant for you to necessarily eat the exact foods listed there every day. However, the fact is, if you follow the exact menu on the foods chart, you will get great results.

For two weeks Denise ate the same kind of food at the same time every day. Sounds crazy, but it was effective. She lost ten pounds in those two weeks. She said she was never hungry, never tired, and never bored (partly because she was focusing on the descending scales, not on the food). At the end of two weeks, I praised her for her resolve and for the wonderful results she had achieved.

But I told her she needed to create variety in her diet, explaining that the foods in the chart were simply examples of how to eat. I told her that her first meal didn't always have to be oatmeal. It could be a whole-grain cream of wheat or a whole-grain dry cereal with soy or almond milk. It could also be a piece of fruit or anything that fits into the calorie count and food category for breakfast. Her second meal could be a hard-boiled egg and some spinach instead of the yogurt and fruit, and so on.

Grasping the principles of the plan

So where did Denise go wrong? When I explained to her the need for variety in her diet, she began to make substitutions that did not meet the criteria established in the plan to assure success. When she attempted to make changes, she did so from a too limited understanding of the principles of the plan. She substituted caloric protein bars for lean meats, vegetable drinks for vegetables, and she allowed her meal portions to resort back to her previous habits of overeating. Because Denise did not immediately grasp the significance of the principles of the plan, her changes compromised the effectiveness of the plan.

For example, week one is to teach you to use the guide as a tool to record your foods; it is not an exact eating plan to follow. Week two is to teach you to record the value of the foods and make some preliminary changes to the diet of week one by altering or increasing foods in specific categories. The primary key to the success of the plan is for you to make slow incremental, easily sustainable changes until you have formed new eating habits. Your long-term success in following the plan is based on grasping the principles behind every change that is being made.

Denise, like so many people, was so desperate to see quick results that she neglected to understand how she achieved her desirable results. In her case, weeks three and four did not show the same descending scale changes of weeks one and two because of her faulty knowledge and unwise changes. However, gradually, her accumulation of knowledge of these principles and taking ownership of the plan laid the foundation for great results for the weeks that followed.

Part of the problem was that Denise, and many other people like her, are slaves to structured routine. Tell them exactly what to eat (the food chart examples) and how to exercise, and they will do it relentlessly. This obsession with structure can be a good thing in some situations of life. For example, it can make you a dependable employee and help you keep your checkbook balanced. But when it comes to eating healthy, exercising, and embracing other positive lifestyle habits, this inflexibility can be detrimental. You need to understand the principles behind the plan as well as the process required for your success.

Taking personal ownership of the process

What I have seen over the last twenty-five years is that unless people/patients take personal ownership of the *process* it's very difficult to maintain newly formed, positive habits in the face of stress and other negative external changes. Trying to follow a plan without grasping the principles of the plan and owning the process it requires is a very shaky foundation for success. Intentionally grasping a good understanding of the scientific basis for the plan (to a certain degree) and the process it requires for success will establish personal ownership for your ongoing health decisions. It will build consistency into your daily decisions, even when the world around you gets stressful.

For example, if I tell you to eat an exact menu for the next thirty days, and you follow the menu exactly, you will lose weight in those thirty days. But if I don't tell you anything about the caloric or nutritional value of the food, or explain the glycemic index of the foods and how to make reasonable substitutions, or the science of spreading out meals or combining your foods for maximum digestion and assimilation of nutrients, or how to maximize your fat loss through strategic timing of when, how, and what kind of exercises to do, you will have no knowledge of the *process* required for your success.

Without that knowledge it is impossible for you to *own* what you did.

You just did what I told you by rote, and because the plan is based on sound principles, it worked. However, because you have no idea about how it worked, it will be impossible for you to sustain the success long-term that you enjoyed after following the plan for thirty days.

I cannot emphasize the importance of this success attitude enough: stick to the plan. No matter if it's my Genesis Diet or another scientifically proven health program, stick to the plan! Resist the urge to make changes based on emotion or personal preference that might compromise the principles of the plan. In addition, be leery of programs that limit your degree of knowledge of how they work. God spoke through the prophet Hosea and said, "My people are destroyed for lack of knowledge" (Hosea 4:6). The more you know about how something works, the better the chances are you will stick with the process.

One final note, do not fret about the changes you are making to achieve your optimal health. Jesus taught us: "Do not be worried about your life" (Matt. 6:25). Simply determine to keep your purpose above your preference.

SUCCESS ATTITUDE #6: FORGIVE THE FAILURES OF THE PAST

Don't bring your failures of the past into the present. Just because a weight-loss plan didn't work in the past or you didn't follow the plan before doesn't mean a new plan, approached with a different attitude, won't work for you now. Sometimes we just need to forgive ourselves for past failures.

One of the most common concerns I hear from prospective patients and attendees of my Wellness Workshops is how the past failures or shortcomings will affect future outcomes. People tell me they tried this, that, and the other thing and nothing seems to work. Some even say they have tried *everything* without success (hyperbole?), so they are convinced there must be something wrong with their metabolism that keeps them from losing weight. Their thyroid is slow or their sugar metabolism is sluggish; that's why they can't get their "couch potato" brain out of the house and into the gym. But the worst excuse is when they tell me that they have tried a program just like mine and it didn't work...those are fighting words!

Justifying the problem

Sometimes people use the failures of the past as an excuse or a means to justify being out of shape and on the potential brink of a health breakdown. Many of these people have convinced themselves that the problem is the program and not themselves, the person. They tried popular weight-control programs and lost twenty pounds, only to regain that weight plus ten after the holidays or their cruise to the Caribbean. They tried the gym but didn't see the expected results. Besides, the machines were always crowded and the classes were scheduled at tough times of the day for them. They went to their doctor of chiropractic for their headaches and felt better after a few adjustments. But six weeks later the headaches came back, and it was easier just to take pain pills.

Of course, in some cases these people have a legitimate complaint; they followed a program, took potions, and did the prescribed exercises, and the results were "no results." The truth is that many wellness programs offer no chance of success, no matter who follows the program. They have no scientific foundation that can accomplish the claims for success. Perhaps the exercise apparatus just doesn't target problem areas or create enough resistance to produce results. The high-protein, just juices, or "eat what you like and sprinkle on the appetite suppressant" diets may sound enticing. But rarely, especially from a scientific point of view, do they create long-term positive and sustainable results. If this is your past experience with weight-loss programs, your concern is easily resolved.

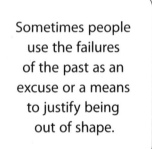

Sometimes people use the failures of the past as an excuse or a means to justify being out of shape.

Forgive the program, forgive the friend who sold you on this "brilliant plan," and forgive yourself for thinking that this shortcut was the key to your "get into shape" solution.

Mirrors don't lie.

For the rest of the folks who have misappropriated their blame for past failures, it's time to point the finger at the person in the mirror, not the plan of the past. For the people who tell me they have tried reputable programs that just didn't work for them…*please.* It is almost a sure thing that the person didn't follow the program exactly the way it was supposed to be followed to achieve success.

Then there is the "I tried a program just like yours and it didn't work" excuse. This used to bug me the most. They don't even know what my program is about, but somehow they linked it to one they tried in the past. These people are the toughest to inform. It's hard for me to convince them of the difference between the Genesis Diet and the program they tried in the past, without creating ill will or leaving a bad impression. Usually I just give them my business card and invite them to visit my website to compare the two programs.

I've also had people tell me, "Doctor V, I'm following your plan and doing everything you told me to do, but I'm not seeing results." Again, they are making the program the problem. When I hear that, I immediately go into my "protect the reputation mode." I ask them, from a knee-to-knee, eyeball-to-eyeball position (this sounds scary, but I'm having fun with you):

- "Are you preparing and eating your foods exactly according to the plan? Let me see your food diaries."

- "Are you doing your exercises every day for the exact amount of time we agreed on? Demonstrate for me now the exercises I showed you."

- "Are you taking your supplements, drinking enough water, getting enough rest, and avoiding unnecessary, self-induced stress, like I told you?"

Their answer 99.9 percent of the time is, "Well, not exactly, Doc." Then I tell them it is time to refer back to Success Attitudes #1, #3, #4, and #5. Your foundation for following a reputable program and succeeding must be your positioning for long-term success as I am outlining here. Only then will you be motivated to overcome spiritual obstacles and embrace attitudes for success that will assure your achieving long-term health goals.

I mentioned the "something is wrong with my metabolism story." The truth is, most of the time their blood work is normal, all scans are normal, and all the stars are exactly where they should be in the sky. What's not normal is their account of their health decisions that day. They forget they ate cookies, and it was ten of them, not three. When they say they exercised every day, they forget that there are seven days in a week, not three. They think that because they went out to dinner one night and the boss bought lunch for them one day, those days really didn't count. The fact is that their metabolism is fine; we just need to work on their memory and their ability to recall the truth.

The bottom line is that if you want to move forward to a healthy future, you have to give up your disappointment with failures of the past. Our enemy, the devil, loves to plant fear, skepticism, and distrust in the hearts of men and women. It strengthens his modus operandi for killing, stealing, and destroying (John 10:10). Making you dwell on past failures is a perfect ploy for him to hinder the growth and potential for your success. The past failures are not there to thwart your progress of achieving your goals; past failures are there to teach you where not to go and what not to do. They direct you, however inadvertently, to the right path where you will proceed with more wisdom than emotion.

SUCCESS ATTITUDE #7: ENDURANCE AND LONG-SUFFERING

When you are focused on getting into shape, you have to face the fact that there will be good days and bad. Sometimes you'll get on the scale and smile; sometimes you'll want to cry. Some days you'll try on those favorite slacks and they fit; other days you can't even snap the button. Some days you'll feel encouraged and empowered; other days you'll want to quit and eat a box of doughnuts. You have to remember to never get too happy or too sad from the report of one day—the short term. It is a matter of developing the virtues of endurance and long-suffering, speaking in biblical terms. If you're sticking with the plan, the results will eventually come, though you may have to endure bad days and suffer disappointments along the way.

Painful progress

Cheyenne got on the scale in my office every week, week after week, and painstakingly watched her weight drop almost imperceptibly: .2 pounds one week, .1 the next, and maybe, if she was fortunate, .3 the next. Needless to say it was frustrating for both of us. And it didn't help when patients scheduled before Cheyenne would come out of the exam room bragging about how they lost 3 pounds last week and a full percent of body fat. Still, poor Cheyenne would pull it together and dutifully come into the office.

Every week we would search her recorded activity to see why she didn't get the results we expected. Cheyenne was neither the super ideal patient nor a covenant-breaking slacker; she just couldn't put it all together. One week she would eat better but have problem getting all her exercises in. The next week the diet was a little off, but her exercising picked up. It took some time, but eventually, with her enduring persistence and perseverance, we established a formula that cleared the way for Cheyenne to achieve her health goals. At the time of this writing, she's losing two or three pounds per week.

No doubt it would have been easier for Cheyenne to quit, given her lack of comprehension and such low positive results. If you face a situation like Cheyenne's, you'll need to decide, as she did, to dig deep and hang on. Quitting cannot be an option. What does it really matter if you take a week, a month, or a year to accomplish your goal? Any positive action you take will improve your overall health. Throwing in the towel can only assure you one thing—a greater chance of getting sicker sooner.

SUCCESS ATTITUDE #8: ACCOUNTABILITY

Accountability is king! Without accountability, the previous seven success attitudes we have discussed have a great chance to crumble. *Accountability* is the success attitude that acts as the glue to hold the others in place, which assures success.

Getting into shape, recovering from an injury, or just trying to drop thirty pounds is no easy task. In the case of Abraham, who was commanded to sacrifice his beloved son, his task was unimaginable. But the attitude and disposition that Abraham exhibited when confronting this task is a classic example of being accountable to God and trusting Him regardless of the hurdles in your path.

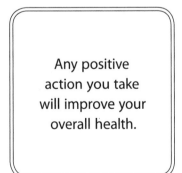

Any positive action you take will improve your overall health.

God desires for us to be healthy and free from infirmity. Sickness that is tied to our neglect or disobedience is a direct offense to the preservation of His temple, our bodies. The task of creating wellness is not easy, comfortable, or convenient, but it is vitally necessary. The success attitudes discussed in this chapter are essential not only to achieving your optimal health goals but also to the achievement of success in every area of your life. Refer to the chart to review the requirements for your success attitudes.

YOUR SUCCESS ATTITUDES

1. Be committed to stop making excuses.
2. When you're convicted to make a change, you must start the process immediately.
3. Be willing to intentionally make sacrifices.
4. Resist the desire to take wasteful shortcuts.
5. Stick to a plan that is proven to work (you don't have to reinvent the wheel) and own it.
6. Forgive and forget your failures, but learn from your mistakes.
7. Be willing to endure and cultivate the attitude of long-suffering. I believe that persistence is omnipotent!
8. Accountability is king! Make yourself accountable to God and others.

ABRAHAM AND THE EIGHT SUCCESS ATTITUDES

In the beginning of this chapter I mentioned that all eight success attitudes were drawn from the account of when the Lord directed Abraham to sacrifice his beloved son, Isaac. A brief summary of Abraham's story will strengthen these covenantal principles in your mind.

#1: No excuse, and #2: Immediate response

> Now it came about after these things, that God tested Abraham, and said to him, "Abraham!" And he said, "Here I am."
>
> —GENESIS 22:1

Getting into shape, for most people, can be a painstaking test and an insurmountable challenge. Abraham was totally accountable to the call of the Lord. When the Lord called, he simply responded, "Here I am." In saying that, he declared that he was ready to do whatever the Lord wanted without any excuses or delay.

In contrast, regarding our call to care for, or in many cases to restore, our physical body, the temple of the Holy Spirit, how often do we respond with excuses, delays, and justifications that declare, "The timing is not right"?

#3: Sacrifice

And then God said something that must have wrenched Abraham's heart:

> He [God] said, "Take now your son, your only son, whom you love, Isaac, and go to the land of Moriah, and offer him there as a burnt offering on one of the mountains of which I will tell you."
>
> —GENESIS 22:2

The Lord challenged Abraham with the ultimate sacrifice. He didn't just challenge him to give up soda or lay off the bread and butter. He told Abraham to give up the very covenant promise that defined his life and purpose. What was Abraham's response? Scripture says that he just got up and went. Without excuses, demanding no explanation, making no argument, he took immediate initiative and was willing to intentionally make this massive sacrifice.

> Accountability is the success attitude that acts as the glue to hold the others in place, which assures success.

#4: No shortcuts, and #5: Stick to the plan

Abraham would go to the exact place God had commanded, a three-day journey with a heavy heart, and stick to the plan God had commanded, no matter how painful:

> So Abraham rose early in the morning and saddled his donkey, and took two of his young men with him and Isaac his son; and he split wood for the burnt offering, and arose and went to the place of which God had told him.
>
> —GENESIS 22:3

Abraham completed the plan God had given him. He didn't deviate from the task, improvise, or compromise it in any way; he didn't bypass or seek a shortcut to achieve the inevitable outcome God had commanded.

#6: Forget past failure, and #7: Be willing to endure suffering

Of course, Abraham did have another son, Ishmael. He was the result of Abraham and Sarah taking matters into their own hands to fulfill God's promise to give them a son. Sarah was beyond childbearing age, so she offered the solution of having a son through her maid, a custom of the day. Did Abraham consider that mistake? If he did, it did not hinder him from going forward to fulfill the command of God in the present. It is touching to witness the trust in God Abraham showed now in the face of this terrible command:

> On the third day Abraham raised his eyes and saw the place from a distance. Abraham said to his young men, "Stay here with the donkey, and I and the lad will go over there; and we will worship and return to you." Abraham took the wood of the burnt offering and laid it on Isaac his son, and he took in his hand the fire and the knife. So the two of them walked on together. Isaac spoke to Abraham his father and said, "My father!" And he said, "Here I am, my son." And he said, "Behold, the fire and the wood, but where is the lamb for the burnt offering?" Abraham said, "God will provide for Himself the lamb for the burnt offering, my son." So the two of them walked on together.
>
> —GENESIS 22:4–8

No matter how bleak the plan looked, Abraham trusted that the Lord was faithful to keep His covenant promise regarding Isaac's becoming the heir of his father's house. Indeed, the New Testament declares that Abraham believed God would raise Isaac from death, if necessary, as long as Abraham stuck to the plan to the end (Heb. 11:17–19). He knew that Isaac was the fulfillment of God's promise and that God could never go back on His word. So he reassured his young son that God would provide the burnt offering, which He did miraculously.

#8: Be accountable

Abraham demonstrated his ultimate accountability to God as he raised the knife to kill his beloved son (Gen. 22:10). In that terrible moment the angel of the Lord called to him from heaven:

> Abraham stretched out his hand and took the knife to slay his son. But the angel of the LORD called to him from heaven and said, "Abraham, Abraham!" And he said, "Here I am." He said, "Do not stretch out your hand against the lad, and do nothing to him; for now I know that you fear God...." Then Abraham raised his eyes and looked, and behold, behind him a ram caught in the thicket by his horns; and Abraham went and took the ram and offered him up for a burnt offering in the place of his son.
>
> —GENESIS 22:10–13

As you meditate on Abraham's obedience, which brought the blessing of God into his situation, consider which of these eight success attitudes you need to cultivate in your heart. God will respond to your cry for help as you identify your weaknesses and determine to let Him transform your thinking to embrace the success He desires for you regarding your health.

MASTERING ACCOUNTABILITY

As I mentioned, I am convinced that, of these eight success principles, *accountability* is the most critical to your success. I also believe it is the toughest of all the success attitudes to master. It is part of our human nature to seek independence and do our own thing. The world has promoted the idea that submitting to authority is a sign of weakness. Some people think that if they show too much dependence on another, it will be misconstrued as feebleness of character. They do not understand the meaning of accountability.

When it comes to helping people achieve healthy lifestyle changes, a patient's accountability is essential for receiving direction, support, and guidance and encouraging proper motivation. My rule of thumb for accountability is this: you must become accountable to someone other than yourself who knows more than you do regarding your health, in this case, and has a vested interest in your success.

"Self-accountability" is only effective for 3 percent of the population.

Otherwise, the "do-it-yourself" accountability is usually the driving force behind the yo-yo diet, the recurrent back pain, and the on-and-off medication roller coaster. It ultimately results in the eventual despair of "it's useless, nothing works for me" attitude. Holding yourself accountable to another person is not always easy, especially if you're not 100 percent convinced of the other person's motive for requiring it.

Before I accept a new patient into my Wellness Program, I make sure I go through with them an exhaustive process of education and indoctrination to assure that every question is answered. I try to position myself as a coach who has a player with great potential to be a superstar. The objective is to groom my player (patient) to physically and mentally become a consistent winner. Patients understand that their results directly impact my professional reputation. This reality creates an environment in which I, as the doctor, become accountable to the patient and his or her overall well-being as well. I guard that accountability by making sure I teach, instruct, and help to motivate them to achieve their goals. The formula is complete with both parties, doctor and patient (or coach and player), having an equally vested interest in the patient's success. In light of this, it is important to remember that getting into shape is not a temporary task; it is a lifestyle transformation that takes months and years to develop and maintain.

Evangelist for accountability

Griselda is one of my star patients and the envy of all the other patients in my Wednesday evening schedule. Every week she lost two or three pounds. This continued month after month, as she never ever gained an ounce or missed an appointment. She first came to my office in a housedress, sandals, and a low-maintenance hairstyle. Five months later, forty-five pounds lighter and 15 percent body fat leaner, Griselda strolled into the office with her skinny jeans, riding boots, and rock-star hairdo. Not only was her physique dramatically different; her overall disposition was strikingly changed as well. Her confidence level had soared, and her self-esteem was at an all-time high.

When conversing with other patients, especially new ones whom she meets in the waiting area, Griselda simply tells them, "Follow exactly what Dr. Vetere tells you. Fill out your food sheets, do your exercises, show up, and be accountable to your appointments, no matter how you feel." Her "evangelistic" fervor cannot be misunderstood because she has the results to back it up.

Your success, after reading this book, is not based as much on the technique and health science that will be taught in the next chapters as it is on your ability to use the knowledge to position yourself for success. That requires that you allow your mind-set to be truly transformed, like Griselda's, to embrace the truth and become *accountable* for your actions, attitudes, and motivation.

Overcoming spiritual obstacles and embracing and adhering to the success attitudes is truly the impetus that will assure your achievement of long-term wellness goals. Your entire success hinges on your willingness to be accountable in the following ways:

1. God your Father and Creator. "Then God said, 'Let Us make man in Our image, according to Our likeness; and let them rule over the fish of the sea and over the birds of the sky and over the cattle and over all the earth, and over every creeping thing that creeps upon the earth" (Gen. 1:26). God created us in His image and likeness and then commissioned us to a great task—to have dominion over all the earth. As Christians, it is our highest obligation to be accountable to God and to respect the body that He has given us and in which He dwells by His Spirit.

2. A doctor or other trained health care professional who is honestly concerned for your overall well-being

3. Those who love you and need you. No matter what your family relationships, if you are wife or mother, husband or father, daughter or son, the restoration of your health is a concern and potential inspiration for others.

Document, document, document

Accountability is always validated by documented evidence. What that means, in the world of getting healthy or losing weight, is that you must record what you do (what you eat, your exercise amounts, etc.) and that you must show your results to someone who cares (the person you're being accountable to) for their approval, correction, and further instruction.

Your willingness to take their advice with a teachable spirit makes being accountable a pleasurable experience for all concerned. I tell my patients all the time, "When you're doing well and feeling strong, I will push you and stretch you to achieve greatest capacity. And, if for some reason you slip and fall, I will pick you up and help you to get straight until you're feeling strong again. Then I will push and stretch you again."

When you succeed, not only does your notebook provide documentation, but also your vibrant health and dramatic changes in appearance will document your success for everyone around you.

This is your appointed time to get your health in order. Please know that I am here to help. My website, www.schoolofwellness.com, has plenty of information and resources, including a listing of doctors who are familiar with the Genesis Diet. As you continue to pursue your health goals, you will be inspired to know that you can actually make changes that last a lifetime.

Chapter 4

MAKING CHANGES THAT LAST

W HEN IT COMES to losing weight and getting into shape, the idea of a fast and easy scientific breakthrough has always captivated the imagination of the shortcut-minded consumer. Science, in its prideful attempt to play God, has misled the public to believe that soon there will be a cure or solution to every health problem known to man. This misleading assumption creates a health care consumer who neglects to make healthy lifestyle changes. They live in the hope that some day in the near future there will be a magic pill, potion, or procedure that will be the instant cure-all for any ill they may suffer.

This sense of false hope has become very problematic to the health care community. Information about disease prevention and healthy lifestyle activities has never been so prevalent and available. There are health-conscious talk shows, radio programs, magazines, books, and, as I have mentioned, hundreds of health-focused infomercials. Health clubs and workout studios are popping up everywhere, promoting specialty niche concepts to satisfy every consumer preference for fitness training.

Yet our nation's increased obesity rate and prevalence of diabetes, heart disease, and many cancers are still on the rise, dramatically increasing the national cost of health care. Some argue that even though the average life expectancy is increasing, our overall quality of life, especially in our senior years, is decreasing. Why? What can be done to change this negative phenomenon?

THE "HOW-TO" KEY TO SUCCESS

In the first three chapters we discussed the *why* for pursuing your personal wellness, possible *spiritual obstacles* that sabotage your efforts, and the *success attitudes* that govern wellness. I firmly believe that if you abide by these biblical principles, you will succeed in any health-related program you choose. Having said that, the next key to your success now becomes the mastery of the process of *how to* apply this knowledge.

In order to make changes that last, your human desire of "I want it now" has to be quelled. Your main focus has to be on changing the destructive habit rather than watching the scale. You must be convinced that lasting results are the product of slow and steady incremental changes in behavior. The change of a habit will have greater long-standing results than any quick and potentially dangerous weight-loss gimmick.

One of the most common questions I hear in new patient consultations is, "Dr. V, how long do you think it would take me to lose twenty-five pounds?" My answer usually surprises them: "What does it matter?" I make these two points very clear to all new patients:

- First, the Genesis Diet focuses on achieving optimal wellness, of which permanent weight loss is a natural by-product.

- Secondly, the premise of the program is that it is more important to focus on long-term fitness habits than to day-dream about the desired beach body.

Our goal is to create a lifelong solution for your optimal health. Once you buy into this philosophy as your primary focus, I have no problem calculating for you an exact date for reaching your goal of losing twenty-five pounds. The point is that your endeavor to master life-changing habits has to become more important than your scale-watching goal. You must understand that achieving your desired weight is only possible when the work required to get there is mastered. Again, slow incremental changes over a long period of time have always been shown to be the most effective formula for achieving success in your health goals.

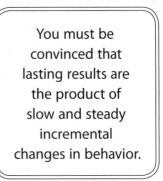

You must be convinced that lasting results are the product of slow and steady incremental changes in behavior.

Alma lost more than twenty-five pounds and got her body fat down just about perfect just in time for her sixtieth birthday. When I first saw her, she was frustrated with her overall health. She was out of shape and burdened by multiple health issues, including terrible back and neck pain. Eight months later, after completing our program, Alma was transformed. She looked great, felt great, and had a terrific new outlook on life in general.

One day when Alma was leaving my office, a woman interested in becoming a new patient was sitting in the reception area. As they passed, I introduced Alma to the woman and asked her to give the woman a word of encouragement. They chatted for a few moments, and the woman asked Alma the typical question, "How long did it take you to lose the twenty-five pounds?"

Alma's response was...you guessed it, "What does it matter?" Then she asked the woman, "How long have you been trying to get into shape?" Her question was a kind way of asking, "How long have you been out of shape?" The woman responded honestly, "Oh, for many, many years." Then Alma repeated, "What does it matter how long it takes? I can assure you that as long as you apply what Dr. V teaches you, and you stick with the plan, you will see results. I can guarantee you that, because I'm living proof that it works. And now I understand that the end results are more important than the time it takes to get there."

Believe me, as a doctor, I'm very sensitive to this time issue that concerns patients. The marketing angle for almost every weight-loss product or service revolves around one of two promises: either "easy to do" or "lose weight in a rapid amount of time." And no matter how many times these program promises "flash and fail," people keep trying them in the hope that *maybe this time it will work.*

ACCEPTING THE REALITY OF THE TIME ELEMENT

If you're out of shape or suffering from an ailment due to poor health habits, you must accept the fact that your poor health didn't just happen overnight. As a matter of fact, most poor health conditions are the by-product of long-term unhealthy lifestyle habits. Sickness is created over months, years, and sometimes decades. Conversely, wellness is necessarily the by-product of long-term attention to practicing positive lifestyle habits. In short, *wellness,* the reverse of sickness, is also created over months and years. Even though this is simply a reality, both physiologically and psychologically, it is not a popular angle for marketing to this "I want it now" society.

The jump-start trap

I have a problem with the jump-start or boot-camp philosophy of starting a wellness or fitness routine. True, it is very enticing to think that you can go from flabby to firm in just ten days. But, for most people, that hope is far from the reality. The thought of correcting months or years of health neglect in just ten days is extraordinarily tempting for anyone to believe. Here are some reasons that these sales and marketing pitches rarely deliver on their promises:

1. The amount of change for the person to make is too overwhelming. Even though the plan may work from a physiological perspective, the average out-of-shape, never-exercising-couch-potato may not be physically or mentally able to follow the plan effectively.

2. The plan itself may be flawed, not practical, or even biochemically dangerous for some people to attempt. People with sub-clinical health conditions such as borderline diabetes or high blood pressure can place themselves at a severe health risk attempting these quick fixes.

I remember talking to a gentleman in the gym who was working out on the elliptical machine next to me. Being a competitive eye-spy that I am, I had to look at his resistance level, speed, and, of course, heart rate. We were moving at the same speed and resistance level, but his heart rate was at 190, while mine was 130. I had to comment to him that I was a doctor and asked if that was his usual heart rate on this machine. That's when he told me he was doing some jump-start program.

I stopped working on my machine (to get his attention) and told him that his heart rate was dangerously high and he needed to slow down now! I could tell by his expression that he thought I was a little crazy. But I didn't want his jump-start program to end with me trying to jump-start his heart after he fell off the machine. What happens much too often is that the "boot camp/jump start" approach to getting into shape leaves the person disappointed and discouraged with the lack of results. Only in certain cases do I believe this approach can be safe and beneficial.

The jump-start exception

Some patients who come to me could be considered "backslidden fitness enthusiasts." They are not in terrible shape, have a history of being in great physical condition at one time, and have no present health issues that would contraindicate a rigorous physical challenge. All they need is a little help with motivation and a whole lot of accountability.

Steven fit this description when he came to my office. He had been in the military, and for years he had lived the lifestyle and knew the meaning of being in great shape. For much of his life the discipline to practice healthy lifestyle habits was built into his job description. Then he retired, and that accountability aspect was missing from his life. Because Steven was used to being accountable to a physically challenging occupation, getting him into great shape again was not a physical challenge; it was more about creating a new focus of *accountability*, that most important success attitude.

The first step was to get him to become accountable to me . . . that was easy. The second and more challenging step was to get Steven to be accountable to himself, but with a twist. Steven was conditioned to focus on taking care of others first. My goal was to get him to understand the necessity of being healthy for himself, his family, and the new opportunities that God was going to give him to serve. Because of his recent lifestyle of fitness, Steven was a perfect candidate to place into a jump-start environment. Once he accepted his new source of accountability, Steven was physically and mentally able to accept any rigorous physical challenge.

Again, let me reiterate that Steven is an exception to the rule for pursuing long-term health goals. Since most people are not like Steven, for whom getting into shape was simply a matter of reviving good health habits, they must accept a realistic time element to systematically be successful, even when "starting from scratch."

Powerful Beginning Motivators

How you view your starting point is critical to your successful journey to good health. Resisting the urge to try to make all the healthy changes needed immediately is so important. Sometimes frustration, guilt, and other negative emotions become the impetus behind starting a weight-loss or fitness program. This faulty motivation is usually problematic to your desired success. The desire to make up for bad choices along with being disgusted at where you are at the moment does not create the proper mental outlook for achieving sustainable results.

Becoming dismayed with your overweight shape or overall level of health is not altogether negative. Your feeling of disgust can actually be quite the motivator if you determine to abide by the eight success principles, understanding that accountability is the most important of those principles. That involves holding yourself accountable to someone other than yourself who is more knowledgeable and has a vested interest in your success. But there is a more effective approach than being motivated by fear or disgust. It could be considered a commonsense approach to optimal health goals.

Identify the cause of poor health habits

Intentionally choosing to improve your health for the future is a wise and commonsense approach to achieving optimal health. The first step in this approach is to identify poor health habits and their cause. People do things habitually usually because, on some level, they give pleasure or help to avoid awareness of pain. That is true even if the habit is eventually destructive.

Simply becoming aware of terrible eating habits, your lack of desire to exercise, and your decision to just take pills to cover up the symptoms of your health problems is not good enough. As I stated earlier, the object is to find out the *why* behind your destructive habits. Why do you eat a certain way, knowing that what you're eating is unhealthy? Why do you sit around watching TV when you can easily go to the gym or even exercise in front of the TV?

Again, let me remind you that, in order to pursue optimal health, you need to take a moment to regroup and analyze yourself spiritually and mentally. What degree of pleasure do you get temporarily from eating rich and tasty food? Is it greater than the pain of getting on the scale the next day? Is the pleasure of loafing on the couch every evening greater than the pain of squeezing into your jeans the next morning?

Even if your emotional or spiritual well-being is battered and you're going through a tough stretch, that is no reason to self-destruct through temporary pleasures of self-gratification. According to the Scriptures, your enemy, the devil, comes in like a flood to destroy you, but God promises that "the Spirit of the LORD shall lift up a standard against him" (Isa. 59:19,

KJV). And Jesus said that the thief comes to steal, kill, and destroy, but He has come to give you abundant life (John 10:10).

It is vital that you keep your spiritual guard up against the enemy's strategies for your destruction. So when you're feeling down and out, or maybe you're just blah about life in general, this must be your cue to get alone with the Lord and reconsider your priorities and change your destructive actions. Sometimes you're not even sure what's bothering you emotionally. But you must still choose to change your actions. As you do, soon enough the cause of your emotional downer will become clear. As you seek the Lord, you will realize that it wasn't so bad after all and that with God on your side you are always victorious. Identifying the cause factor for your poor health choices will help you to recognize what triggers your destructive behavior.

Become conscious of stress triggers

Once you identify those emotional stresses that trigger your poor lifestyle choices, the next step is to analyze your reactions. If there are distressing problems at work or relational issues going on in the home, the object is to be conscious of how you attempt to counteract the pain of those problems. Again, the goal of human nature is to avoid pain. When that is not possible, the next best thing is to escape pain through some *immediate,* though temporary, *pleasure.*

In order to maintain optimal health in the face of pain, your great task is to intentionally bypass that desire for immediate pleasure. Instead, you need to take actions that will result in lasting healthy pleasure. As a Christian, you need to make choices that reflect God's character, not those that conform to the destructive actions of the world. As you turn to the Lord, He will give you the strength to make the healthy choices. We have His covenant promise that "with God all things are possible" (Matt. 19:26). No matter if you have never attempted to get into shape or if you have been struggling to do so for years, when you turn to the Lord, He will give you a strategy and the divine help you need to make your plan successful.

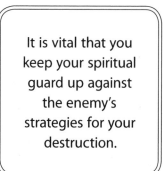

It is vital that you keep your spiritual guard up against the enemy's strategies for your destruction.

Cultivate small beginnings

We can learn from Jesus's life how He approached phenomenal changes that would have eternal worldwide impact. When He came to earth, He didn't attempt to change the world all at once. He didn't set up worldwide speaking engagements, nor did He go right to the top rulers and try to convince them of His mission to revolutionize the world. Jesus's life ministry was relegated to a few square miles; He intentionally kept His "organization" to twelve men, and He didn't address an influential political ruler until the day before He died. His life epitomized the reality of small beginnings. So, what was His plan of action, and how does that relate to your getting into shape?

In His divine wisdom, Jesus obeyed His Father's instructions to choose a few men who would follow Him. Their lives would be transformed through that relationship. Even though Jesus's ministry of healing and miracles impressed the multitudes, He focused most of His teaching and character transformation on His disciples. These few simple men, transformed by their love for Christ, would eventually exert such eternally sustainable persistence in preaching the gospel of their risen Lord that they would influence the entire world forever.

This concept of starting small and being empowered to multiply your results exponentially can be applied to your pursuit of optimal health. Instead of trying to make every change that is needed immediately, identify the lifestyle change that would be the easiest for you to make right now—one small beginning that would cause the least amount of stress and disruption to your current behavior habits.

For example, instead of trying to go completely vegan (eating nothing but vegetables, herbs, and fruits) tomorrow, just add an extra salad per day to your diet. Or choose to drink one less soda a day and one more glass of water. In later chapters we will discuss a more exact plan, but the point I am making is that for achieving long-term health goals, it is imperative that you attempt to make the easiest and simplest changes first. These small beginnings give you the opportunity to feel the satisfaction of being successful and inspire you to move on to more challenging changes. Small incremental successes build momentum to empower you to attempt greater challenges and enjoy greater success. When this concept of beginning small is practiced over an extended period of time, you will see the development of a new and sustainable health habit for life.

This is true even if you hit a roadblock at some point in the plan. No one is perfect, and there will be times when you fall into a slump. Even the greatest baseball players are not exempt from falling into a batting slump. They can go weeks without getting a hit, and then all of a sudden they get one hit and their hitting gets back to normal. The same can happen to you in your journey to getting into great shape. I normally go to the gym four or five days per week, but occasionally things happen and my schedule is turned upside down. Occasionally I find myself having to verbally motivate myself to get back into gear.

Sometimes your lazy, complacent, subconscious mind kicks in and tries to tell you that you deserve a break: enjoy a piece of cake today and hit the gym again on Monday. That's when you should use the old cliché, "Today is the first day of the rest of your life." Every new day is a potential new start or in some cases a restart. Remember, always start with small sustainable changes and know that the big changes are soon to come.

> Small incremental successes build momentum to empower you to attempt greater challenges and enjoy greater success.

"Drag a buddy in" plan

One of the most common practices among people attempting a fitness, wellness, or weight-loss program is the "drag a buddy in plan." People think that if they get someone to join the gym with them or go with them to the weight-loss meetings, the buddy system will assure accountability and eventual success. In some cases this may be true. But more likely, if you become dependent on someone who is not completely committed to sticking to the plan, you can possibly be setting yourself up for failure. On the other hand, I have seen the buddy system work really well when the relational "chemistry" is right. I've had couples and groups as large as five people do the Genesis Diet together with great success. In these cases I have observed certain tangibles in place that promote their success.

- One person finds exercising easy and holds the other person accountable to exercise, while the person who is not keen about exercising is quite disciplined in preparing healthy food choices. This combination of the strengths of one person offsetting the weaknesses of the other contributes to the success of both parties.

- One person, perhaps a highly motivated mom with her kids or a boss who rounds up a few of his subordinates to join him on his quest to excellent health, can create a group dynamic that works.

I have seen both of the above scenarios work well for all involved. If you're thinking of getting someone to join you in the Genesis Diet or any other program, make sure that the "chemistry" is correct for motivating you toward success. If you have to convince someone by twisting his or her arm to join you, I can assure you that plan is destined to fail.

Another option for accountability partners is to join a program or a fitness club that has group participation sessions. Most health clubs have a variety of training classes where you can meet people. The "be a friend make a friend" philosophy can prove to be very effective in this situation. The Genesis Diet includes weekly education workshops, which are also a perfect setting for those who are interested in the "buddy system" to meet others with like-minded goals.

In selecting a buddy, it is vital that you avoid people who have the tendency to put you down or who reflect a critical spirit, jealousy, malice, or envy. Be sensitive to the people who are around you. People who support your desire to achieve your health goals will let you know right away through their actions and words. Those who can be a hindrance will also be obvious in the same way. They can be members of your family, fellow employees, and yes, unfortunately, church friends.

Regardless of the opinions of those around you, learn to hold your plan sacred and let your results speak for themselves. I've had patients complain to me about how their family is no support to them. I understand that some patients may be exaggerating just to get my sympathy, but you do need to avoid family conflicts that threaten your success. In a sense, you need to be selfish and focused on yourself to maintain your goals.

For example, you may need to buy and cook your own food, watch TV in another room, and do your exercise routine while you watch your favorite show. Sometimes, negative input from family members means they want to see you fail because they don't want you be better than them. They are content in their poor health habits, and as the saying goes, "misery loves company." You will have to separate yourself from those negatives and focus on relating more to those who support you in your goals.

It will take discipline to make these tough decisions, especially if you are a very social person. Friends and coworkers may invite you for lunch or occasional parties. You don't want to seem antisocial or rude, and you don't want to be perceived as a fitness elitist. So be prepared to suggest places to eat where you can get a healthy salad.

> Learn to hold your plan sacred and let your results speak for themselves.

You could also tell the host of a party that you will be there but will be eating before you arrive and ask them not to be insulted. Let them know you appreciate their hospitality, but that your health goals are of vital concern. Real friends will fully understand and more than likely encourage you. As you can see, there's a lot more to getting into shape than just joining the gym and buying a bunch of vegetables. Preparing for the emotional, spiritual, and even social challenges is essential for the success of your journey toward optimal health and lasting results.

Chapter 5

THE SCIENCE OF LOSING BODY FAT

I F YOU HAVE diligently read the first four chapters, you will understand how important they are to the information in this chapter. However, if you just opened the book to this how-to overview for getting into shape, I urge you to start reading from the Introduction and through the previous four chapters before trying to implement this plan. I cannot stress enough the importance of understanding the correct mental and spiritual attitude as the basis of being successful in the health plan presented in these next chapters. Knowledge is great, but knowing how to properly execute it is critical for success.

In this chapter I have included the specific topics relating to wellness that are relevant to your success in getting into great shape. As we discuss each area and how it relates to your health goals, I will explain why the measurement of your body fat percentage is important. I like to use it not only as a barometer for tracking your fitness progress but also as a tool to augment my patient recommendations. In later chapters we will discuss specifics of these topics in implementing your personal fitness plan.

EVALUATING FOOD INTAKE

Food intake is the most obvious topic for virtually all weight-loss/fat-loss and wellness programs. The first concept to understand is that everything we eat or drink has to be measured in calories. I know that all the trendy and cutting-edge weight-loss programs like to shy away from counting calories, treating it like it's some archaic practice from 1905. But whether or not you count calories, just continue reading to see that they are secretly being counted for you. The bottom line is that your intake of calories must be counted.

Understanding your energy source

All food (or drink) that you consume that has the ability to supply energy to your body has a caloric number. That means that the food or drink must contain carbohydrates, proteins, or fats in order for your body to use it as an energy source. Each food category, when broken down into its simplest form through the digestive process, will then be transported by blood vessels into the liver for processing and detoxification. The liver then prepares the simple sugars (primarily glucose), amino acids (from the proteins), and lipids (from the fats) to be disseminated into the bloodstream to supply energy and repair to the body.

A properly balanced diet, which we will discuss later, will supply the correct amount of glucose for active energy use along with the correct amount of proteins and fats for organ/gland repair and regeneration. A diet with an overabundance or deficiency of certain food groups will lead to biochemical chaos that will result in glandular and organ breakdown, excessive fat storage, and overall chemical imbalance. In short, this biochemical chaos "creates" the overweight person, who is likely to get sick prematurely.

The ability to gain weight or to lose weight is primarily controlled by the intake of food *calories,* not food *volume* or quantity. Later you will understand how critical this fact is to the plan for eating all day and still losing weight and body fat. In order to properly measure the number of calories you need to consume to be successful in your health plan, it is necessary to calculate your BMR (basal metabolic rate). That is the key information needed to gauge the amount of calories that are necessary for you to gain, lose, or maintain weight.

Your present BMR is equal (approximately) to the amount of calories you burn during the day while you are *at rest* or just being alive. Your metabolic rate obviously increases with the activities and physical demands of your day. The simple science behind the formula is that consuming less food calories than your BMR will result in weight loss; consuming more food calories than your BMR will result in weight and fat gain. So, whether or not you want to count calories or have someone else count them, have no fear; your body is counting them. Their total count will be reflected in the exact ounces of weight lost or gained.

Calorie defined

What is the definition of a *calorie*? Webster's dictionary states that a *calorie* is "the amount of heat (or energy) required to raise the temperature of one kilogram of water one degree Celsius."[1]

You may be wondering, "So, what in the world does raising the temperature of water have to do with the number of calories in the bagel I had for breakfast?" That is a fair question. When applied to food, a calorie refers to the amount of energy or heat the food can produce or store, based on the volume or weight of the food. It also refers to the amount of heat or energy the body has to produce to burn off a gram of protein, fat, or carbohydrate.

Confused? Don't be. Let me explain, using the example of your bagel. The average bagel contains about 270 calories, primarily from carbohydrates (starch or sugars). Eating this bagel will give you 270 calories of energy. That means, in order to burn off the 270 calories from eating the bagel before they are converted to fat, you would have to generate the heat or energy necessary to burn that many calories. That would be calculated to thirty minutes on the treadmill or twenty laps in the pool. Thinking in reverse, in order to run thirty minutes on the treadmill, you needed to fuel up, like putting gas in your car, with enough calories to give you the energy to complete that thirty-minute task.

All calories are not created equal.

You also need to understand that all calories are not created equally; that is, all foods are not created equally with respect to calories. Foods are assigned a caloric number based on the amount of energy necessary to burn off 1 gram of the particular food category to which they belong.

For example, it takes 9 calories to burn 1 gram of fat and approximately 4 calories to burn 1 gram of protein or carbohydrate. The mathematical conversion for grams (for those of us who still can't figure out the metric system) is 1 ounce is equal to approximately 28 grams. So if you eat a bagel that is 68 grams of carbohydrate (2.5 ounces) it will give you 270 calories (4 x 68) to use as energy. Four ounces of solid protein is equal to 112 grams, which would mean 448 calories.

So why does my calorie counter say my 4-ounce grilled chicken portion is only 120 calories? Because when the fluid is removed (if you were able to dehydrate the chicken to just the protein value), it would probably be equivalent to only 1 ounce. Furthermore, different meats, beans, and other proteins have varying amounts of inherent fluid and density that will alter their exact protein weight, hence, their caloric value.

Lastly, there are the fats, which are rarely consumed on their own. They are part of fatty foods like bacon, which is still 50 percent protein. This can really complicate the mathematical formulas (grams of fat multiplied by 9 grams of protein multiplied by 4, less any water content). That's why there are standardizing laboratories to measure these numbers. For simplification, all you need to do is look at the package label or go online and search for "number of calories in 4 ounces of grilled chicken," and you'll get the answers you need to record your caloric intake.

In addition, most foods are a combination of carbohydrates, fats, and protein. However, there is no need to carry a calculator and a scale with you every time you go shopping or eat in a restaurant. After measuring your food portions once or twice (see chapter 6), you'll have a good idea of what a cup of food is or what 4 ounces of chicken looks like on your plate. Since you probably eat the same menu of food each week 80 percent of the time, memorizing that a cup of cooked broccoli (and most other solid vegetables) is 20 calories is not too difficult. Just in case, it's not a bad idea to bookmark a calorie counter site on your computer for easy reference.

The glycemic index

Another point of interest in the food intake category is the science of the glycemic index (GI). There are a few diet programs on the market that state they work with the "science" of glycemic index as a means for losing weight; these diets are based on a valid premise. Simply defined, the glycemic index of a food is based on how fast the food you eat turns into sugar available in the bloodstream. The standard measurement is based on the time it takes for simple sugar to be present to a certain degree in the blood.

Foods that consist mainly of simple sugar like cakes, white breads, white rice, pasta, and cereals usually have a high GI. Foods that consist of more complex carbohydrates such as vegetables, whole grains, and most fruits have a lower GI. Foods that consist of little or no carbohydrates have a very low GI. Most health experts agree that eating foods with a lower GI number (50 or below) provides great health benefit, while consistently eating foods with a higher GI (60 or above) can lead to health issues. I recommend that you bookmark a GI list on your computer also.

Let me explain how this GI number works. Its application will help you make substitutions from less healthy foods to more healthy foods as you progress in your health plan. Low GI foods like whole-grain brown rice, spelt, barley (not whole-grain cereal or bread), and vegetables consist mainly of complex carbohydrates. It takes the liver longer to convert whole grains to available simple sugars (glucose). In addition, the liver releases the sugars at a slower rate over a longer period of time.

So what's the health benefit? The longer it takes for carbohydrates (sugars) to be released into the bloodstream, the less danger there is for them to spike the blood sugar level. That means the pancreas has to work less, not having to release sudden and large amounts of insulin as for simple sugars. Less stress on the pancreas is good news for diabetics.

Also, the slower the sugar enters the bloodstream, the less likely it is for the insulin to store the sugar as lipids in fat cells. This storage process is a big reason why people who eat lots of foods with simple sugars gain weight. Giving the body sudden, large amounts of simple carbs raises the blood sugar level to above normal. The body's only response is to get the sugar out of the bloodstream by producing more insulin to convert it to a lipid and store it in the body's fats cells. Fat cells swell, and you gain weight!

Another health benefit of foods that are lower on the glycemic scale is that they are high in fiber, low in fat, and filled with nutrients. They are also lower in calories and more filling. When God designed the garden, He had the perfect menu for mankind in mind; fresh fruits, vegetables, beans, and legumes are an ideal combination for complex carbohydrates, lean proteins, and essential fats.

SOME NOTABLE MYTHS

- Diet sodas and foods with artificial sweetener help you lose weight: Wrong. Many researchers are discovering that these sweeteners actually can cause you to consume greater levels of other high-sugar foods.

- Low-fat foods help you lose weight: Not always. Just because a food is low or no fat doesn't mean low sugar or low calories. Nonfat ice cream or brownies may be low in fat but still high in sugar. Also, fat is not the main reason you gain weight; weight gain is caused by an overconsumption of sugar.

- High-protein diets help you lose weight fast: Sometimes, but most of the time at a high health risk. High-protein diets are slow to store fat and have the ability to turn off the hunger response faster than other diets. The lack of dietary carbs forces the stored fat to break down faster to supply the body with glucose for energy. This approach may have some short-term weight-loss benefit, but the disruption it causes in normal function, the unavailable nutrients from the other food categories, and the production of toxins and acids from the high proteins can lead to an eventual metabolic disaster.

THE SCIENCE OF EXERCISE

Exercise is probably the most loved thing people hate to do. We all know its benefits, we know its importance for keeping our cardiovascular system healthy, and we wish there was an easier way to get it done. I mentioned in chapter 3 that the shortcut exercise routine is the most sought-after component in the world of fitness. To make the science of exercise more complicated, there are literally dozens of different categories, types, and styles of exercise. It's no wonder people are confused. Yet the scientific truth remains that you must exercise on a regular basis in order to enjoy good health.

I believe that the wide variety and different styles of exercise are a good thing. When I go to the gym, there are some people working with weights, others using the aerobic equipment, and others taking one of the studio exercise classes. Having a favorite type of exercise is a good thing because it will keep you engaged and decrease the chances of your dropping out. One of your most important tasks is to find a style of exercise that produces real fitness and that you have fun doing.

Before I discuss different kinds of exercises, I want you to think about what kind of exercise (dance, running, or playing a sport) you would be happy to participate in. For example, my wife likes to work out on the elliptical machine—not necessarily for the function of the machine, but she likes the TV that's connected to it, especially from 7:00 until 8:00 p.m., when she can watch her favorite shows and trade her workout time for 600 calories burned. In contrast, my assistant does an hour of Zumba dancing with her little granddaughter. The baby soon becomes exhausted and falls asleep, and my assistant gets in her afternoon workout in peace. I go to the gym and pretend I'm twenty years old again, playing two or three games of full-court basketball. It beats the boring treadmill except for the bumps, bruises, and other assorted injuries that result from the mind and body not being the same age.

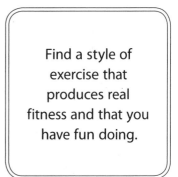

Find a style of exercise that produces real fitness and that you have fun doing.

Finding an exercise system that is fun for you will keep you engaged, even when you don't feeling like working out. In the next chapter we will discuss a specific formula that will help you to create a fundamental exercise routine, which is both fun and effective. In this wellness program you will learn to implement the following kinds of exercise into your daily wellness routine.

Strength training

The concept of strength training is to build bigger, stronger muscles. This is usually achieved when you do fewer repetitions working with heavier weights. The science for strength training is to overload the muscle to the point that the muscles fibers are actually torn. This sounds rather dangerous and unsafe. Without supervision, it could be harmful. When done correctly, your body's amino acid repair system rebuilds the muscle bigger and stronger than before.

In addition to building stronger muscles, strength training helps drop the percentage of unwanted body fat. Again, this can be dangerous if done incorrectly or recklessly, so make sure you have a trainer or training partner who knows what they're doing to help you. Even if you have done this type of training before, always be careful and realize that weights and machines have no mercy when handled without caution.

That being said, I highly recommend that everyone in my Genesis Diet program engage in some level of strength training. You will learn that I am a big fan of mixing up and changing exercises to avoid getting into a rut. Never get into a boring physical routine. Not only will you lose interest, but also it will not give your body a chance to acclimate to specific workouts that lead to muscle adaptation.

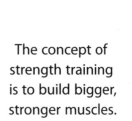

The concept of strength training is to build bigger, stronger muscles.

Aerobic training

Many people, especially when they first start an exercise program, gravitate to one or more of the aerobic training machines at the gym. I am not saying that you have to join a gym or buy expensive equipment to have a great aerobic workout. In the next chapter I will show you that all you need for a powerful workout are your legs and a two-by-four-foot space; I will exhaust you in four minutes.

The purpose for aerobic training is multifaceted. It's a great way to tone muscles, burn fat, and increase the strength and output of the cardiovascular system. Monitoring your aerobic fitness level requires measuring your heart rate, time elapsed, and calories burned during your routine. This monitoring can best be done when using professional, gym-grade equipment. But there is also some high-tech equipment available for less than one hundred dollars (and the size of a watch) that can monitor your progress. Even a brisk walk and a wristwatch to monitor your heart rate will do the trick. Simply completing the exercise routine in chapter 6 will get your heart rate up significantly.

Of course, you need to heed the classic disclaimer to check with your family health professional before you do any kind of exercise. Remember, the purpose of this book is to motivate and empower you to get started toward new health goals and to maintain your program. But don't be foolish and do something to hurt yourself. Not only would that be a terrible outcome for you, it would not be a good plug for book sales. (I just had to say that.)

Muscular endurance training

The definition for *muscular endurance training* may vary slightly among trainers, but I like to give my patients the following explanation. Remember that strength training involves low repetitions with heavier weights. In contrast, muscular endurance training involves higher repetitions with lighter weights until you achieve muscle exhaustion. The goal is to train the muscle to stay strong over a long period of time. It is also great for fat burning and cardiovascular toning.

Of all the types of weight training, endurance training is usually the safest; it is also the most rewarding the next day. That is because, although you will be sore the next day and realize that you have worked out, you will not be as debilitated as you would if you had an aggressive, straight workout.

Muscle flexibility

You got it…stretching! Stretching is notoriously neglected in the world of fitness training and sports. This is especially true for men who think they have to get right to the weights or tie their sneakers and jump onto the basketball court. I believe that a large portion of fitness-related injuries could be prevented if people would just spend the time needed to stretch before and after their workouts.

I can give you all the scientific proof of the benefits of stretching. But because many people are "crisis learners," they have to wait for their own injury before learning those benefits. Like everything else related to good health, stretching has to become a habit. In the morning when you wake up, before you get out of bed you need to stretch for two to five minutes. This also applies to pre-exercise and post-exercise routines; you need to spend two to five minutes stretching each muscle group you intend to exercise.

The main benefits of stretching are to increase the range of motion of both the muscle and joint as well as to increase blood circulation to the area being trained. Increased range of motion minimizes the chance of muscle pulls or tears. The increased blood supply warms the muscle and avails it of needed oxygen and glycogen (stored sugar in the muscle used for energy) for maximum performance. Stretching after a workout promotes healing and recovery time for maximum muscle gain from your workout.

This is not crisis-based knowledge; it is the understanding needed to exercise wisdom in maintaining your healthy workout.

Power training

Power training is a little more advanced than the previous styles we discussed. It is more designed for competitive athletes. However, I encourage all my patients to try to incorporate some of this exercise style into their workouts.

The technical name for this type of exercise is *plyometrics* or *functional exercising*. Athletes use this type of training to improve the speed and power of muscle performance by rapidly increasing the neuromuscular response. What I like about this style of exercise is that you can generate a lot of intense work in a short period of time. Plyometrics training can be done with most muscle groups of the body. Granted, some of the maneuvers are easier than others, and for a few of them you need to be in great shape before trying them.

A basic power-training maneuver can be performed as a modification of a lunge exercise. The simple lunge is performed by taking a three quarters step forward with one leg. Then bend the back leg, dipping your body and bringing your knee straight down toward the floor. This movement will cause the knee of the front leg to bend naturally. This maneuver results in engaging practically all the muscles of the legs and buttocks. Repeat the maneuver, stepping forward with the opposite leg to train both lower extremities equally.

To turn this exercise into a power-training exercise, you would jump between dips and switching legs. For example, step forward with your right leg and bend your left leg, pointing the knee straight down. When reach the bottom of your lunge, jump up and switch legs in the air, landing in a lunge position with your left leg in front of your right. This may sound too acrobatic for some, but as you improve your fitness level, the only way to improve your overall fitness is to increase the challenge of your exercise routine. Power training can be incorporated with other leg exercises and upper body training as well. On our training website are several videos you can view to see these exercises in action.

Importance of cross-training

This overview of various styles of exercise emphasizes an important aspect of your fitness plan: *cross-training*. I am a strong advocate of cross-training to help prevent *muscle adaptation*. Using the same exercise or workout routine continuously allows your muscles to adapt in a way that they use less energy to perform the same exercise. The object of cross-training is to never allow your muscles to use just one type of exercise for a long period of time. Muscles have to be challenged in order to maximize their performance.

Regardless of the type of exercise you choose, you must appreciate the covenantal design of muscle function. God designed your muscles to be rigorously used. You dare not abuse them to the point of irreparable damage or leave them to atrophy, which aids fat gain. Muscles that are regularly exercised, by their very design, increase their function, tone, strength, speed, power, and overall longevity. Strong, well-toned muscles also diminish fat gain and improve overall physical and mental wellness.

In short, physical fitness enhances every part of your physical being, which is the temple that God uses to get His work done in the earth. We clean our churches, repair the pipes, and paint the walls. We sometimes give money to the church building fund to repair the roof, even if we have a leak in our own roof. We make a commitment to the maintenance of our church building. In that same way, if you want your building—your body—to stick around in good working order, then make a commitment to its maintenance; no more excuses.

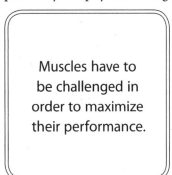

Muscles have to be challenged in order to maximize their performance.

Valuing Water and Rest

Drinking plenty of water and getting your required rest are critical elements in the overall formula for optimal wellness. I can give you all the benefits of these two vital aspects of health, but, sadly, simple facts don't always motivate people to do what is most beneficial. In addition, the purpose of this book is not to flood you with research data, hoping that you adopt this logical, nonemotional approach to life.

Healing hydration

Most people are simply interested in *results*. In that regard, there are some interesting facts about how drinking water will increase your desired results of losing weight and dropping body fat. Drinking water in order to be properly hydrated is critical for normal cellular function, especially for the liver and for skeletal muscles. Let me explain.

The liver is responsible for controlling a large portion of overall fat metabolism. Dehydrated liver cells (lack of water) have diminished function, which slows down this important process. It also slows down with the conversion of sugar into available energy, the storage and release of vitamins, and the overall detoxification of the body. In short, water supports the liver's ability to improve your metabolism.

The same is true for your muscles. Well-hydrated muscles perform significantly better than muscles less hydrated. The ability of the muscle to convert sugar to energy, replenish amino acids for muscle growth, and remove toxins for muscle recovery are all based on maximizing the hydration of muscle cells.

Some researchers have found that drinking 16 ounces of water a half hour before each meal may aid the weight-loss process.[2] The physiological reasons are not clear, but people in these test studies have lost weight. The working theory is that the increased water raises the speed of the metabolism, increases the activity of the liver and kidney to promote proper detoxification, and lowers the body's desire for excessive sugars. My only caution is not to have too much water while you are eating. This can neutralize the enzymes and other digestive acids in your stomach and small intestine, which may lead to improper digestion of food and assimilation of nutrients.

Recovery through rest

Getting enough rest has a multifaceted impact on weight loss as well as weight gain, not to mention your overall health. Proper rest is critical to supply the time necessary for the body, especially the muscles, to recover from the stresses of the day. During rest there is diminished fluctuation in heart rate, metabolism, and hormonal release. These conditions are all conducive for cellular recovery and repair. Muscles that have been recently stressed (exercised) have time to recover, rebuild, and gain maximum function.

On the other hand, lack of rest leads to physiological and emotional stress. Sleep deprivation studies show that people who experience inadequate rest suffer severe lapses in judgment and the inability to execute tasks, especially those that are willpower related.[3] This discomfort becomes the perfect recipe for emotional or binge-related eating. Stressed people, deprived of normal willpower, usually resort to destructive, "feel-good-for-the-moment" eating habits, with little regard to the consequences.

Getting enough rest is like any other task you need to complete in your day. If you want to maximize your body function and avoid the chaos of an "I didn't get enough sleep" day, make intentional plans to get to bed earlier, even if you have to miss your favorite show.

UNDERSTANDING STRESS AND WEIGHT GAIN

You may be aware that stress is a major factor in the unhealthy progression of gaining weight and increasing body fat levels. It is also a driving factor behind every major catastrophic disease. The obvious reason for its impact on your health is that when you're stressed, you have no time to eat properly and no time to exercise. As a result, your meal choices revolve around fast foods and high pleasure snacks. Instant gratification and the desire to "feel good" overshadow the sensible preparation required for healthy food choices.

Learning healthier responses

Giving in to your bad habits of emotional eating and your lack of motivation to exercise are just temporary fixes for battling stress. Actually, this typical reaction to stress is more of a *learned* response than a psychological reaction. So, with the right coaching, it is possible to learn a healthier response to stress that has positive outcomes for your health. For example, when you are under stress, if you turn to rigorous exercise as opposed to rigorous eating, the results will be very positive. Exercise stimulates your pituitary gland to release *endorphins*, hormones that have the ability to block the transmission of pain signals in the nerves. In addition, they create a generalized state of euphoria that simply makes you "feel better."

The biochemistry factor of stress

The greater factor that causes stress to impact weight gain centers more around *biochemistry* than emotional response. When you are faced with a stressful situation, like a close call on the highway or running into a suspicious character in a dark alley, your body has a natural hormonal response system designed to provide physiological help in a time of need. In lay terms this response is called the "fight-or-flight" mechanism.

When your mind perceives the stress of imminent danger, your brain releases a series of hormones in association with direct neurological stimuli that immediately cause your adrenal glands to flood your bloodstream with adrenaline and cortisol. These two hormones have a powerful impact on the function of the body.

Adrenaline, also known as epinephrine, will increase your heart rate and overall cardiac output. It also facilitates blood flow to your brain and skeletal muscles and increases accessible blood sugar levels by converting glycogen (stored form of glucose in the liver) into available glucose. In essence, this hormone produces the energy to run, fight, or use muscular action on an extreme level of intensity and duration that would be impossible through normal physical action.

Cortisol, the other major stress hormone, is released from the outer layer of the adrenal gland. In a high-stress encounter, cortisol targets fat cells to release lipids that are then converted to available blood sugar. In the event of a high-stress crisis, massive amounts of glucose are needed to supply the muscles with the necessary fuel to handle such a prolonged and strenuous event.

My "flight" crisis

On the Thursday following the attack of 9/11 on our nation, I joined a team of clergy to help in the relief efforts at Ground Zero. The enormity of the situation was complicated by the safety instructions that were given to all present. The engineers were not sure about the stability of the surrounding buildings, so they set up an alarm system to warn the workers in case of a pending structural collapse. At the moment we entered the work area, that alarm blasted.

Without thinking, I just started to run and run and run. I ran until I almost passed out. My heart was racing, and I could not stop shaking. It took almost forty-five minutes for my heart rate to return to normal. Thanks to my body's fight-or-flight mechanism, the amount of adrenaline that flooded my bloodstream must have been enormous.

Remember, the release of these hormones in a high-stress situation is natural, normal, and potentially life saving. Besides being released during a flight-or-fight crisis, these hormones are naturally released at a lower rate during the day to regulate many metabolic functions in the body. For example, adrenaline works antagonistically to insulin to regulate blood sugar levels. Insulin, a hormone released by the pancreas, creates a passageway for glucose to enter tissues cells, which is necessary for normal cellular metabolism. Insulin also facilitates excessive blood glucose being stored in the liver and skeletal muscles as glycogen; through a series of chemical conversions it stores lipids in fat cells.

In a normal situation, the pancreas would produce slightly more than enough insulin, creating an eventual healthy drop in blood sugar levels. When the hypothalamus perceives this drop in blood sugar, it produces its hormone, which stimulates the pituitary gland to produce a hormone, which finally stimulates the adrenal gland to produce just enough adrenaline to cause the glycogen in the liver to get reconverted back to available blood sugar. This precise combination of insulin and adrenaline is critical for the regulation of normal blood sugar levels

Cortisol also has normal non-stress related functions. It is important in the maintenance of normal blood sugar levels. It does so by stimulating the creation of glucose from all three food substrates: carbohydrates, proteins, and fats. Cortisol also works as a natural anti-inflammatory in the event of injury and infection and as an antihistamine in the case of allergic reactions.

So how does emotional stress affect your biochemistry to make it conducive to weight gain, fat percentage increase, and make you vulnerable to other health conditions such as diabetes, heart disease, and cancer? When you're faced with a fight-or-flight crisis, your neuroglandular system naturally engages. Heart rate increases, muscular function elevates, and excessive glucose is generated to supply the need for "superhuman" energy. That is meant to be a *temporary* response.

In your daily life, when you are faced with emotional stress, the same mechanism kicks in, except without the need of elevating your heart rate, heightening muscular contraction, or releasing excessive glucose. Continuous emotional stress, such as ongoing family problems, financial challenges, job-related tension, etc., keeps your adrenal glands continually releasing abnormally high levels of both adrenaline and cortisol. This condition is harmful to your health.

The problem is that there is no need for the fight-or-flight response. These excessive amounts of adrenalin and cortisol, not used up as they would be in a crisis, are promoting the metabolism of fats and proteins in certain areas of the body and redistributing fat stores in the abdominal region. To complicate the matter further, the increased blood sugar levels now stimulate the production of insulin, which promotes more fat storage and a subsequent drop in the blood sugar. As a result, normal sugar metabolism is altered, and tissue cells begin to crave glucose. Now, the consumption of fast high-sugar junk food becomes the perfect solution.

Ongoing problem

The above scenario is just the beginning of the biochemical disaster that continual emotional stress produces. Continued high levels of adrenaline will eventually affect the arterial walls in the blood vessels of the heart, brain, and retina of the eyes. Unrelenting neuromuscular contraction of the muscles around the spine can lead to vertebral subluxations, which then leads to neurological interference of spinal nerves, resulting in pain and a plethora of other organic and glandular problems. But it gets even worse. The unnecessary fat metabolism caused by the high levels of cortisol creates an abundance of dangerous free-radical molecules, which can damage cell membranes and even cause damage to cellular DNA. The result of this damage is associated with every chronic and debilitating disease, including the big three—heart disease, diabetes, and cancer.

So when someone says, "Take it easy, or you're going to have a stroke," they're not kidding. Some stress is avoidable, and some is not. We will discuss ways to eliminate stress in chapter 10. For now, it is important that you learn to identify what is triggering your emotional stress and begin to visualize the damage that's occurring on the inside of your body. This understanding may be enough motivation to help you call on God, trusting His covenant promises that He has a plan for your life and that He will always lead you to safety.

> "For I know the plans that I have for you," declares the LORD, "plans for welfare and not for calamity to give you a future and a hope."
> —JEREMIAH 29:11

Those who wait for the LORD will gain new strength; they will mount up with wings like eagles, they will run and not get tired, they will walk and not become weary.

—ISAIAH 40:31

Come to Me, all who are weary and heavy-laden, and I will give you rest.

—MATTHEW 11:28

PREPARING FOR YOUR WELLNESS PROGRAM

In this overview of your wellness program, we have discussed the major *why* factors that, if not properly addressed, can have negative consequences on your wellness goals. Failing to take ownership of these issues will result in unhealthy weight gain, prevent weight loss, and negatively impact your overall health. The principles discussed in these first five chapters are giving you the knowledge you will need to apply as you begin your journey to getting into great shape.

Applying this knowledge concerning food intake, exercise types, and stress-related biochemistry may seem a little over the top for some readers. But, assuming that you are determined to get into shape and stay in shape, you will soon realize how valuable this knowledge is. Sustainable habits can only occur by taking ownership of knowledge that is relevant to your goals. That is what I call the *why* principle. If you don't know why you are doing something, it becomes impossible to do that "something" consistently over a long period of time. The hope of enjoying the benefits of healthy lifestyle habits should be enough motivation for most people to stay in shape. Remember, it's those benefits received by applying knowledge that will encourage you to get healthy.

Encouraging success story

My friend SR was a sixteen-year-old high school basketball standout who developed severe, unrelenting knee pain. An examination, confirmed by an MRI, showed that he had a partial tear in his anterior cruciate ligament (ACL). The exam also revealed that he had a torque imbalance of the pelvis and a subluxation of the sacrum, which caused one of his legs to appear shorter than the other. The imbalance in the pelvis and leg lengths had caused an abnormal stress on the knee joint, eventually leading to the tear in the ACL.

Surgery to repair the ligament would be the obvious medical option, but that would mean sitting out the current basketball season on the bench. He feared that the college scouts would soon forget who he was, and those who remembered him would surely not forget the "player with the knee surgery." The other treatment option was to balance the pelvis and sacrum with an aggressive frequency of chiropractic adjustments, apply therapeutic procedures directly to the knee to promote healing of the tissue, and give SR a rigorous program of stabilizing and strengthening exercises. SR and his dad opted for my suggestion to treat/correct the problem naturally.

The basketball season would begin in four weeks, so we needed to work hard. Every time I saw SR, I explained and demonstrated to him the purpose, rationale, and goal of each of his exercises—the *why* factor. He asked questions and did the exercises in front of me to make sure he was doing them exactly right. His coach called me to say that SR was doing his exercises, stretches, and other balancing techniques more diligently than any player he had ever seen.

The happy ending to the story is that SR was back on the basketball court in less than three weeks, pain free and playing great. Instead of having to watch the season from the bench, scouts will be watching him on the court. The key to SR's success was his motivation. For SR, the benefit of getting a scholarship and playing college basketball outweighed the tiresome and tedious hard work of doing his exercises and keeping his chiropractic appointments. He made sure he did every exercise and procedure exactly the way I showed him. He listened diligently and learned the rationale behind the exercises he was doing and the chiropractic adjustments he was receiving. SR received the benefit of a healthy knee, without surgery, because he applied the knowledge he was taught.

SR is an example of the power of understanding the knowledge and science of what produces wellness. Whether your challenge is pain, injury, or being overweight, when you understand how the physiology of your body functions, it's hard not to visualize the harm of eating certain foods or other poor lifestyle choices. Understanding and applying the *science* of getting healthy and dropping body fat is critical for your success. So get ready; it's time for the Genesis Diet school.

Chapter 6

THE GENESIS DIET AND EXERCISE FORMULAS

I N THIS CHAPTER you will begin to understand why the principles we discussed in the first five chapters are necessary to your success for long-term wellness. Having made a commitment to those principles, your goal now is to explore a step-by-step process that will lead you safely on your journey to optimal health. I have taught this process to hundreds of patients who have succeeded in reaching their health goals.

Before we get into the logistics of the program, let me encourage you that wherever you are in your health walk is *where you are*, and that's OK. You don't need to put extra pressure on yourself because you are more out of shape than you think you realized; don't be down on yourself because over the last couple of months you have really "let yourself go." There may be a negative driving force telling you that it's too late to get into shape or that you're too far gone.

Your goal may be to lose ten pounds or one hundred pounds. Maybe you're hoping to avoid the diseases of your ancestors, or you're trying to eliminate the need for your diabetes or blood pressure medications. Regardless of your personal health goals or the underlying motivation for improving your health, now is the time to begin that journey. And where you are is the perfect (only) starting place.

YOUR PERSONAL STARTING LINE

The first task at hand is to accurately determine the numbers for your weight, body fat percentage, and basal metabolic rate (BMR). Your BMR is the amount of calories you are burning in an average day that results in maintaining your current weight and body fat percentage. This reality check is important to determine your personal starting line. Don't be tempted to jump the gun and create your own daily calorie target amount.

Understanding basic diet factors

Your body is very scientifically sensitive. It responds to how you eat, when you eat, what you eat, the amount you eat, and the combination of food groups you eat. These factors are all critical to maximizing the quickest, safest, and overall healthiest way to get into shape and achieve maximum wellness. Dropping your calorie intake to 800 because you read about some celebrity who did it by drinking a weight-loss shake and eating a slice of pizza every day is clearly not healthy. That is an obviously unsustainable wellness plan.

Determining the first three numbers you need for a starting point—weight, body fat percentage, and metabolic rate—can easily be determined if you have a special scale that measures all three components. Otherwise, getting an accurate body fat percentage and metabolic rate can be somewhat challenging, but it can still be done with a little work. You can do a search on your computer to "calculate body fat percentage" and "calculate metabolic rate or BMR." There are dozens of sites with calculators that will figure these numbers for you. They will ask you questions about your height, weight, age, and gender to help formulate the numbers you requested. Also, you will probably need a tape measure to measure the distance around several different areas of your body.

While this method may not be the most accurate, it will give you a basic starting point. Ideally, I would suggest that you invest in a digital scale the records all of these numbers. The cost of these scales has gone down significantly over the years. (I use a Tanita brand digital scale. It is very accurate, and I have had no problems with it for years.) Once you have these baseline numbers as your starting point, you can determine your daily target calorie intake.

Remember, your goal is to lose as much body fat as you can, as fast as you can, and as safely as you can, using a scientifically sound approach. (Please check with your personal physician or health care provider before beginning this fitness program.) Science has determined that to lose one pound of body fat requires burning 3,500 calories.[1] My experience also says that reducing your daily calorie intake by 1,200 calories per day is practical for most people, as long as the total daily target calorie intake does not drop *below* 1,200 calories per day. For most people, an intake of less than 1,200 calories per day can actually slow down your metabolism and detrimentally affect the biochemistry and hormonal balance in your body.

Applying the numbers

Mary weighs 200 pounds with a body fat percentage of 45 percent and a BMR of 2,900 calories. That means on any given day, Mary needs to eat 2,900 calories to maintain her 200-pound body weight and 45 percent body fat. If we eliminate 1,200 calories from her daily diet, her new target calorie intake goal would be 1,700 (2,900 − 1,200 = 1,700). This goal places Mary well within a safe range for reducing calories and boosting her metabolism with exercise to lose a pound of body fat every three days.

Jane, on the other hand, weighs 140 pounds with a body fat percentage of 36 percent and a BMR of 1,950. If we eliminate 1,200 calories from her daily diet, her new target calorie goal would be 750 (1,950 − 1,200 = 750). This number is too low for optimal success. At 750 calories a day, Jane may lose weight, but she will also slow down her metabolism and compromise other health aspects of her body chemistry.

Typically, people like Jane who allow their caloric intake to drop below 1,200 daily will lose weight steadily for the first couple of weeks and then plateau after that. In addition, the stress created on their glandular system to adapt to these severe metabolic changes can weaken their immune system and leave them susceptible to a wellness breakdown. In other words, they will increase their chances of getting sick. To avoid this unhealthy scenario, proper exercise is essential, which I discuss below.

In summary, your goal is to eliminate 1,200 calories daily from your diet, if possible, without dropping below a minimum of 1,200 calories as your daily caloric intake. In Jane's case, she cannot decrease her caloric intake by 1,200, especially when she adds exercise to her routine.

Factoring in exercise

Unfortunately, reducing your caloric intake alone will not result in the lowering of your body fat percentage. Eating less calories and making healthier choices of foods not only cause Mary's and Jane's weight to drop, but doing so also *lowers their metabolic rate*, which *slows* the weight-loss process. In order to avoid this downside of a slower metabolism, both ladies will have to increase their exercise program.

To really lower her body fat, with a daily caloric intake of 1,700 Mary will need to burn at least 300 calories daily in her exercise routine, which will help her maintain a steady level of weight loss (1,700 − 300 = 1,400). For Jane, the maximum daily caloric intake she can eliminate is 750 to maintain a daily target intake goal of exactly 1,200 calories. That means to reach the differential of *eliminating* 1,200 calories daily for sustained weight loss, she needs to burn 450 calories (750 + 450 = 1,200). Her exercise routine will need to be at a level to burn 450 calories a day to be on a track for losing one pound every three days.

From her baseline numbers, it is obvious that Jane is in better starting shape than Mary. Because Mary is heavier and has more body fat, she can eliminate 1,500 calories a day through diet and exercise, which means she can lose weight at a faster rate than Jane. However, Mary has a lot more weight to lose than Jane, which means that Jane will probably get to her weight-loss goal sooner. In addition, Jane will reach a point where she will actually have to begin to *increase* her food intake along with increasing her strength training exercises to maximize her eventual ideal body fat percentage.

The point is that whether your starting point is like Mary's or Jane's, or somewhere in between, you need to understand that there is a weight-loss/exercise *formula* that works for your particular situation. And that formula will keep changing as you progress toward your health goals in order to keep your metabolism functioning optimally to meet your weight-loss goals.

Understanding the Food Diary Log

The Food Diary Log is an important factor of the program designed to guide you into eating a balanced proportion of calories correctly from various food groups throughout the day. This plan is important to maximize sugar metabolism, promote the development of lean muscle mass, and assure that you will never be hungry. (See Appendix A for a sample Food Diary Log. You can also download the Food Dairy Log from the www.schoolofwellness .com website.)

In the first column, you record the time of day you eat your meals or snacks. This column serves several purposes. First, it gives you a visual understanding of your eating pattern:

- What foods you like to eat and when

- How much you eat at what hours of the day

- How you spread your meals over the course of the day

- Times you consistently skip meals

Second, it gives you information about how you handle stress as well as an idea of your time management. Was it a rough day, and cookies for dinner seemed appropriate? Were you running behind schedule, and the fast-food drive-through solved the problem? At first your Food Diary Log is used simply as a diagnostic tool to figure out problems in your time-related eating habits. Eventually it becomes your tool for correction, modification, and accountability to help you reach your wellness goals.

The second column on the log is to record the number of meals you eat. This column is just a space holder. It doesn't mean you have to eat six meals per day. I just use it as the place to separate times when you eat. We will discuss later why the ideal eating pattern is six meals during the day, spreading out the meals every two hours.

The third column is the food breakdown column. Here you will need to be very accurate and detailed. The objective is to record exactly what you ate and its volume. For example: 8:00 a.m.: 8 oz. of oatmeal with ¼ cup of skim milk. An incorrect recording of the same meal would read: a bowl of oatmeal. This entry is inadequate because a bowl really has no measurement. How big is a bowl? The difference in 8 ounces of oatmeal and the amount that fits in your favorite cereal bowl could be as much as 150 extra carbohydrate calories. Also, the entry does not include the ¼ cup of skim milk. Just because you always put milk in your oatmeal don't mean its calorie count is not separate from the oatmeal. Although skim milk may only be 20–25 calories, a few calories here and there add up at the end of the day. The point is, *everything counts.*

The next six columns are the food group calories count sections. These are generalized sections where you record the amount of calories for the category of food you ate.

- C: carbohydrates in the form of starches and grains

- P: proteins in the form of meats, beans, eggs, and nuts

- V: vegetables, excluding those that are high in carbohydrates such as corn and potatoes

- F: fruits and berries

- D: dairy, which is separated from the general protein family

- BO: butter and oils

You will need to be as accurate as possible in recording the amount of calories that corresponds to the food you ate. Sometimes this can be straightforward and simple, but sometimes it can seem complex and confusing. The point is to remember that this is a guide to give you direction. In the case of that 8-ounce cup of oatmeal, the recording of the calories is clear and easily measurable. The box says the serving size is 8 ounces and the calories for one serving are 150. Oatmeal is a carbohydrate, so you simply record 150 in the box that is under the C.

Because some foods are a combination of food groups, they can be a bit more challenging to record. Soup, stews, breakfast bars, and pizza are a mixture of different food groups, but don't panic. It's fairly simple to resolve. (Please see Appendix B for helpful tips for counting calories.)

Calculating calopoints

To make the math easier, I tell my patients to omit the last zero of the number of calories, making it a two-digit number (e.g., 150 calories is the same as 15 calopoints). This makes it easier to add later on.

Remember, the objective for recording the calories in the food columns is not to test your patience, mathematical skills, or ability to tolerate tedious tasks. You will see that it is simply a guideline to manage your calories by category and determine your total calories to maximize your weight-loss efforts. Eventually you will commit many of these calorie counts to memory, making the process easier.

The last three columns of the Food Diary Log are for recording the amount of water you drank ("W"), the number of calories you burned during exercise ("E"), and a reminder to take your daily supplements ("S"). They are very helpful to remind you not to miss any of the elements of your wellness program.

At the bottom of the log is the space for totaling your daily calories eaten from each food group. These totals will give you a general idea of the amount of food you're eating in the various food categories at the end of the day. Quite often people are shocked to see how many calories they have consumed in specific categories. The most common "awakening" is usually the amount of carbohydrates people consume. I have found that most people who are overweight usually unknowingly consume many more carbohydrates than they should.

The last grid on the bottom of the log is for recording the target goals and target percentages of food categories established for your weight-loss program. I usually start patients off with a goal of 30 percent total calorie consumption of carbohydrates and proteins, and a 10 percent total consumption of the other four groups: vegetable, fruit, dairy, and butter/oil. Occasionally these amounts are modified for the patient with certain health conditions such as diabetes or for someone who plans to engage in vigorous muscle-building exercises. However, the above formula works well for most people who want to lose body fat and regulate their body chemistry.

Look at the completed Food Diary Log below. The 1,200-calorie (120 calopoints) diet breaks down into 360 calories for carbohydrates, 360 calories for proteins, and 120 calories for each of the vegetable, fruits, dairy, and butter/oil food categories. It might help if you view each of these food categories as "bank accounts" that you do not want to overdraw.

Completed Food Diary Log

Total daily calorie intake for patient's wellness program: 1,200

	Calories	Calopoints
Total from carbohydrates	360	36
Total from proteins	360	36
Total from vegetables	120	12
Total from fruits	120	12
Total from dairy	120	12
Total from butter/oil	120	12
Total calories	1,200	120

The carbohydrate and protein accounts

Assuming your total caloric intake cannot exceed 1,200 calories, your goal for your carbohydrate bank account, which is mainly made up of grains and starches, is to keep that number less than 360 calories (36 calopoints) daily. There is no exact science to explain when consuming too many carbohydrates in a day starts causing the formation of excess lipids, which are stored as unwanted fat. But the fact is, it happens. A good starting point for your carbohydrate intake is 30 percent of total daily caloric intake (360). If you stay at that number or below and notice that BMR and weight are dropping, more than likely that is the correct number for you at present.

Later in your program, when your fitness level changes, these percentages may also have to be adjusted. The same is true for your protein bank account. The objective is to stay at or below the 360 daily count. The exception to this protein number would be when the level of exercise increases; then the calories from certain proteins should increase to satisfy the demand to replenish amino acids for muscle growth.

The vegetable account

The vegetable account is probably the most critical for people who are trying to drop pounds and body fat. Our society is notorious for consuming huge amounts of dead foods. These are the processed carbohydrates and proteins with little nutritional value. Vegetables are God's natural food source filled with life-giving nutrients, fiber, water, essential fatty acids, and vast untapped healing properties.

Most patients, especially the big folks, tell me during our initial consultation that they love vegetables and that they eat tons of vegetables every day. I always find it amazing that they would actually think I believe their story. How can you be 100 pounds overweight and eat "tons" of vegetables at the same time. I call this "selective delusionalism"—my phrase.

The lettuce and tomato on the half-pound burger is not a salad. French fries are not vegetables, and the sauce on your pizza is not a serving of tomatoes. Another example of selective delusionalism is the 2 cups of spinach you ate, forgetting to mention it was creamed spinach, which is 60 calories of spinach and 300 calories of creamy butter sauce.

Consider the huge amount of vegetables that 120 calories represents for the average person, especially for the vast amount of people who hardly have any vegetables on a daily basis. Six cups of salad and 3 cups of cooked mixed vegetables add up to 120 calories of vegetables. For many people this is the difference maker. This shear volume of vegetables may be close to the total volume of all foods they're used to consuming in any given day; yet vegetables have very few calories.

The fruit account

For many people the fruit account is similar to the vegetable account. Very few out-of-shape people reach their target fruit goal of 120 calories on any given day. Again, the people suffering from selective delusionalism may argue the point, citing the few slices of apple pie and a quart of fruit juice they consume. But the scale will always prove them wrong.

The optimal goal is to eat the whole fruit, especially those in which the skin is edible. This assures the best opportunity to receive the nutrients and fiber that God originally built into the fruit. Of course, some fruits have greater nutritional value than others, and some are significantly higher in sugar than others, so managing your fruits is very important.

For example pineapples are nutritious, taste great, and are wonderful for promoting proper digestion. But pineapples are also high in the glycemic index and have more calories per cupful than other fruits. This can be a red flag for some people, especially diabetics, or for patients just trying to stay under 10 percent for their fruit intake. If you love pineapple, a good idea to enjoy this sweet fruit without harm is to cut it into small pieces and mix it with your salads or vegetables, or even use it as a garnish with your meats and fish. It adds a flavorful twist to your meals, and its enzymes help with the digestive process.

In short, the overall goal is to reach the fruit account number or at least come close to it. At least you will be eating a food source that is more nutritious, higher in fiber, lower in fat, and lower in calories than any sweet snack man can manufacture.

The dairy account

For your optimal wellness plan, the dairy account is a take-it-or-leave-it account. Personally, I'm not very fond of dairy products, not for any other reason except that they have little nutritional value. The protein in most dairy is not easily digestible, the nutrients are usually diminished or denatured through the pasteurization and homogenization processes, the fat content is usually too high and unnecessary, there is no fiber, and the calorie count is usually enormous compared to volume.

The main nutrients dairy products supply, vitamin D and calcium (the old marketing strategy), can readily be found in most leafy green vegetables, citrus fruits, and a walk in the park on a sunny day. In addition, I have seen many patients improve their immune function and respiratory function when they eliminated dairy from their diet. The proteins in dairy can also create allergic reactions that precipitate asthma, other allergies, and frequent ear infections. And, of course, there are many stomach and bowel conditions associated with the lactose.

If you have to have dairy in your diet, you must try hard to stay under the 10 percent allotted daily amount. There is one partial exception to this rule: yogurt. The protein in the yogurt is digestible because of its content of bio-friendly bacteria. As a result, yogurt can be a somewhat healthy treat, snack, or breakfast alternative. That is not true, however, if you choose yogurt that the manufacturer tries to make too delectable by adding sugars, nuts, chocolates, and sweetened fruits.

The butter and oil account

This account, like dairy, is also not a "have-to-reach-the-goal" account. Butter and oils to enhance the taste of foods and for cooking should be used in moderation, keeping a keen eye on the amount so that you do not exceed your account limit. The 10 percent or our 120-calorie limit is easily reached; one pat of butter and a tablespoon of "heart-healthy" olive oil, and you're over the limit.

THE FOOD DIARY LOG IN ACTION

As you make long-term, healthy lifestyle changes to reach your immediate health goals and be able to sustain them, your purpose for monitoring these food category counts becomes clear: to track your eating habits and train yourself to stay within the account limits. At the beginning, most people will realize they are exceeding their limits on their carbohydrate and protein accounts while falling dreadfully short on their vegetable account. Cultivating the habit of writing down what you eat, when, and the quantities you consume breaks the selective delusionalism syndrome and gives you an injection of reality of what you're really eating on a daily basis. Many people believe they can simply recall everything they eat at the end of the day; I assure you I have seen that practice fall very short of accuracy. The simple act of writing down what you eat will make you conscious of what you're putting into your mouth.

As part of the protocol for my patients, I review the Food Diary Log on a weekly basis. This is the only way to develop accountability, put correction into action, and develop a strategy for success. Given this avenue of accountability, many patients begin to limit their food intake just because they can't believe they are eating so much. It also helps them to know they will have to show me their Food Diary Log at the end of the week.

At first you learn to use the log as a guide to help you make corrections in your food choices. Substituting fruits for other sweets. Trading a cup of rice for a cup of veggies to cut down the carbohydrate count. Grilling the chicken and baking the fish instead of frying them. Eating one pat of butter instead of two. Cooking your oatmeal in water instead of milk. Happily, the end result is you will eat all day, never get hungry, increase your energy levels, and lose weight every week.

These actions are the beginning stages of becoming accountable for your health goals. Actually, by the time you master the practice of managing your calorie count and food portion habits using your written log, you don't have to write it any more. You have established the knowledge and habits you need to sustain your health goals.

As always, success is a result of slow incremental changes over a long period of time. The objective in learning the food managing and correct eating process is to develop a healthy sustainable habit, which is unaffected by external stresses. True, the process may be tedious in the beginning. You may think that following a commercial weight-loss menu or ordering weight-loss food online may be an easier, less strenuous alternative. My experience has been that the sustainability factor for those weight-loss options is close to zero.

As I mentioned earlier, taking ownership and understanding the science (to a certain degree) of your health goals will absolutely give you a greater sense of purpose and stronger motivation to fulfill them. It is your personal application of these principles that greatly increases your success rate. Recording the information is all about developing accountability habits. In the end, you know that transformation of actions must first begin with the transformation of how we think.

TIMELY EATING FOR OPTIMAL HEALTH

One of the most effective health innovations in the past thirty years has been the management of diabetes. However, it is not based on new breakthrough medications or the potential science of stem cells developing into insulin-producing cells. It is a simplistic model of *adjusting food intake* as a means to regulate blood sugar levels. If a diabetic is able to regulate blood sugar through dietary means, he or she will decrease the chances of physiological damage caused by spiking blood sugar levels.

Unfortunately, the average overweight, out-of-shape, high-body-fat-percentage person who is not yet diabetic may not feel concern of developing the disease. But if they continue their lifestyle of spiking blood sugar, it will surely result in continued rapid fat gain and, eventually, to a problem handling blood sugar: diabetes.

The premise behind recording the time of day that you eat is partially to get an idea of what you are eating and when. It is also a gauge for how far apart you are spreading your meals and how much you are consuming at each of those meals. I encourage you to analyze your eating patterns in light of the following problematic patterns. Then consider the ideal pattern of eating for optimal health.

The big breakfast, late lunch, big dinner scenario

Some people just enjoy eating a big breakfast. The justification is the fantasy that they want to start the day off with a lot of food so they can have energy for the rest of the day. In addition, the typical school system, which has a long way to go before it catches up with the USDA's current food pyramid, erroneously promotes the high-carbohydrate, high-calorie breakfast as a way for our children to charge their day. In reality, the big breakfast filled with empty calories from simple sugars and fats actually *dis*-charges their day, setting them up for metabolic turmoil. Instead of increasing energy by eating a big breakfast, their body is constantly trying to regulate blood sugar levels affected by all those calories.

Here's what happens. In the morning when you wake up, your blood sugar numbers should be at a very stable level. As you begin to move and get ready for your day, your physical activity requires glucose, causing the blood sugar levels to drop. This combination of an empty stomach and lowering blood sugar levels triggers the hunger response. That metabolic light bulb goes off and tells you to sit down and eat.

Here's where habit overrules chemistry. If your meal is significantly high in calories, especially from carbohydrates, the natural biochemical drop in blood sugar you experienced earlier is much smaller than the massive influx of sugars you are getting from your big breakfast. In very short order, your meal will create a huge surplus of glucose that is being pumped into the bloodstream.

Because your activity level when you first get going in the morning is usually minimal compared to the activity that occurs later in the day, that surplus of sugar needs to be removed from the bloodstream. So, your pancreas kicks out insulin and begins the arduous task of getting the glucose out of your bloodstream and storing it in your liver and muscles. However, most of that excessive glucose will be converted into lipids and stored in fat cells.

In addition, the adrenal glands produce adrenaline (as we discussed earlier) that will attempt to regulate the eventual resting blood sugar levels. They also produce the cortisol (which is naturally highest in the mornings upon waking) that redistributes fat to the abdominal area. This process is the perfect scenario for a depletion of energy instead of an energy boost.

As the scenario of the big breakfast continues, the person is not hungry for a while afterward. They allow six or seven hours to pass before eating their next meal. In the meantime, after their body recovered from the stress of the big breakfast and subsequent regulation of glucose, the blood sugar begins to creep down again. But now the person doesn't have the time to stop and eat. They delay their next meal, but their body doesn't get it.

When the blood sugar drops from lack of intake, the adrenals kick in to get the sugar back up. Besides this fluctuation in hormones, the body naturally starts slowing down the metabolism because, for all it knows, it may never get another meal. So it goes into conservation mode, causing unnecessary hormonal changes that redistribute body fat and can even alter the person's mood. The automatic drop in metabolic function also slows down the body's ability to lose weight and burn body fat. By the time the next meal comes, the person's whole metabolic balance has already been thrown off.

Finally, to finish off this already chemically chaotic day, this person decides to eat a big, hard-to-digest dinner. This untimely high intake of calories creates a similar dilemma for the body to that of the big breakfast. This evening meal will create an even greater propensity to gain weight, because at night the individual is less active and will soon be in bed. This inactivity forces the body to store a majority of the blood sugar from that meal as fat instead of the needed glycogen in the muscles and liver.

The no breakfast, big lunch, late dinner scenario

This is a common scenario with the "I'm too busy to even breathe person." Typically this person wakes up in the morning and is immediately in a rush. Everything is a blur. Wash up, fix hair, put on clothes, a quick look in the mirror, and then out the door with not a second to spare. Every day is the same routine, rush and run with no time for something so time consuming as breakfast. Waking up earlier and having clothes laid out the night before would be way too inconvenient. This rush mode is just another habit that needs to be modified.

On the other hand, there are a number of people who say they are just not hungry in the morning. Being hungry, for them, is a relative term. They may not be hungry upon awakening. But if they planned their morning time and activities better, there is good chance they might change their mind before they left the house. In both cases, not always being in a rush and intentionally planning morning time more efficiently would definitely create an environment for consuming some food before the day starts getting real busy.

Regardless of the reason for not eating breakfast, the subsequent physiology still comes into play. As I mentioned, when you first get up in the morning, your activity level is relatively low compared to what it will be later in the day. Your blood sugar levels are comparatively normal, so not eating immediately would not create a great metabolic deficit. But not eating for several hours after awakening can create a physiological problem.

Harm in skipping meals

Sometimes dieters think that if they skip a meal, this decrease in calorie consumption should translate into weight loss. Actually, the result is quite the opposite. In the case of missing breakfast and waiting five to seven hours to have your first meal, you are actually creating a situation for your body to gain weight. As you go through the morning hours, your blood sugar will steadily drop. The more time that passes, the more your blood sugar will drop, which signals to your body to begin to use its stored reserves of blood sugar from the liver and muscle glycogen. As we discussed before, the adrenal hormones stimulate the release of these sugars in an attempt to regulate the blood sugar.

Concurrently, the innate intelligence of your body recognizes this change and lowers your overall metabolism to conserve energy. You know that sooner or later you're going to have a meal, but your body has no idea that it will receive more nutrients. So, the longer you wait to eat, the slower your metabolism functions. Suffering long periods between meals can actually cause the body to promote muscle catabolism, which is the breaking down of protein for energy use in an unhealthy way. Fat catabolism can also occur, breaking down fats for energy, but not in a way that would be healthy for getting in shape.

Another problem occurs when you skip breakfast and finally eat a meal, especially a large one. Remember, you woke up, rushed around, went to work or school, and now, six or seven hours later, you decide to eat. You say to yourself, "I'm starving." In reality you are not. But physiologically, your body thinks you are. That is why it slowed down your metabolism to conserve nutrients.

Now, your "I'm starving" mentality drives your food selection and volume. You crave foods with high carbohydrates. The hours of food deprivation cause you to believe you deserve a reward of "super tasty" food. At the time you eat that meal, your metabolism has slowed way down. Your body is in complete conservation mode, focused on reserving energy.

You eat your big meal with tons of simple carbohydrates, hard-to-digest-proteins, and unnecessary saturated fat. The liver is inundated with sugars, fats, and proteins that need to be processed. Some of them are stored in the liver itself, but most are released into the blood as part of normal physiological function. However, the demand for these energy resources is low because of your slowed metabolism. So the body begins to store much of these calories into fat.

Of course, the body will replenish its cells and tissues with needed nutrients, amino acids, and essential fats. But the slower metabolism at the time of consumption greatly promotes the storage of fat. Also, as your body tries to digest this large meal, blood supplies are drawn to the digestive system away from the muscular and neurological system. Your body's attempt to digest the meal and normalize blood sugar levels actually creates the dreaded "post power lunch" fatigue syndrome.

Once you begin this cycle of events, it's hard to stop the process. Your blood sugar levels will stay high for a while with the unnecessary abundance of stored energy your body is attempting to regulate. As a result, you may not be hungry for hours, which often promotes the late-night dinner effect.

The high-carbohydrate breakfast, no lunch, big early dinner scenario

After reading the previous scenarios, you may be aware of where this eating scenario is going. The large high-carbohydrate breakfast generates an abundance of energy resources during a time of day when there is really not a need for them. This eating pattern typically is simply an eating habit; it is not a biochemical necessity. The increased glucose gets converted and stored as fat, your energy level soon drops, and the vicious cycle that we discussed in the previous scenario proceeds.

From a healthy metabolic and biochemical perspective, these three eating scenarios establish a powerful argument for the necessity of eating timely meals throughout the day. As a doctor, when I see eating habits recorded on a Food Diary Log, it gives me a clear picture of the patient's eating habits and a possible reason for his or her inability to reach weight-loss and body-fat goals. The ultimate goal should be to space your eating times from two to two and a half hours apart six times a day.

Your goals is to eat your biggest meals during the busiest time of your day when you need the most energy, reducing the quantity of later meals as the demand for energy in your day decreases. This timely eating allows incoming blood glucose to be used for the greater energy demands at the present time while diminishing the chances of spiking sugars levels and the unwanted storage of fat. In addition, the consistent influx of food resources for your body provided by eating more often reduces metabolic stress, chemical fluctuations, hormonal imbalances, and personal energy levels. When you combine timely eating with better eating habits and food choices, you will begin to see tremendous changes in your overall physical and mental well-being.

Late-night eating

Late-night eating creates its own set of problems, especially for the person who is unconscious of health issues. The later you eat and the larger amounts you eat, the greater the metabolic stress on your body chemistry. At the end of the day, your metabolism naturally begins to slow down. Your need for glucose and other nutrients is diminished, and your body is looking to stabilize its blood sugar. The late dinner, especially one of large quantities of hard-to-digest foods is most problematic. Going to bed with a full stomach, with no real energy demands for an influx of blood sugar, can do nothing but cause the body to store fat as you sleep. Definitely not part of the Genesis Diet model.

And it's not over yet. By the time you wake up, your metabolism can still be in fluctuation. If this is typically your eating habit, your sugar levels will still be a little elevated, and your desire for a morning meal will be reduced. If this is typically *not* your eating habit, your body will work aggressively to attempt to regulate your blood sugar, creating a low blood sugar situation that generates an increased morning hunger response.

The holiday nemesis

Many times these out-of-control eating scenarios happen during holidays. You may have fairly decent eating habits, but once the holidays come, you tend to get out of control. You find that you are hungrier than usual, you eat large quantities of high carbohydrates, and a vicious cycle sets in. I can't tell you how many times I've heard the complaint, "I was good with my eating until the holidays came. I don't know what happened; I just lost control." That's partially true. It was also the fact that you created a physiological cycle with strong chemical reactions because of eating increased quantities of food at the wrong times.

ADJUSTING FOOD TYPES, CATEGORIES, AND AMOUNTS

As I mentioned earlier, it is critical that you be accurate when recording the type and the amount of food you are eating in your Food Diary Log. This will help determine the calorie amount of each food and help you make sensible substitutions based on glycemic index and other factors. Also, in association with the time of day column, you can begin to adjust meals to help manage blood glucose needs during active and inactive times of the day.

Remember, your goal is *to make slow incremental changes over a long period of time.* Initially, your exercise is just to record down whatever you eat. After doing that, you need to assign calorie numbers to each of your foods in the associated columns with a goal of staying within your calorie limits for each food group. Finally, you need to fine-tune your food choices to create the maximal dietary benefit.

During the first few weeks of implementing your plan you may notice that you have no problem reaching your carbohydrate and protein limit, but getting to even half your vegetable limit seems impossible. Then you start implementing some of the techniques of the program, and before you know it, eating 120 calories of vegetables is just a daily habit. Using the substitution technique will also help. For example, eating brown rice instead of white rice, using stevia instead of sugar, and drinking herbal tea instead of coffee are all sensible substitutions. Sometimes you will have *taste* and *texture* issues when substituting foods, but they can be conquered over time.

Also, categorizing the foods correctly when you record them is very important. For example, beans, even though grown in the garden, are placed in the protein family, not the vegetable family. Eggs, even though they are found in the dairy section of the supermarket, are also in the protein family. You will learn how to juggle the food categories to allow more flexibility in your meal planning; especially in the beginning, it is better to be as accurate as possible, learning to put the correct food in the correct category. The main purpose is to ensure you receive the proper nutrition that each category can offer.

Your goal is wellness.

Remember, your goal is wellness, not just weight loss. You can choose to eat only green vegetables all day every day, without including beans, nuts, legumes, grains, potatoes, or corn. You will lose weight eating that way, but you will also lose muscle mass and be deficient in other nutrients like essential fatty acids, which are necessary for normal cardiovascular and neurological function.

At the end of each week a quick look at the Food Diary Log will help you pinpoint:

- Food choice problems consistently occurring at specific times of the day

- Areas where you can substitute a better choice in food type or preparation; for example, oatmeal instead of sugary cereal; grilled chicken instead of fried chicken

- Times of the day or events that occur at work that alter or obstruct your plan

- Obstacles that seem to be out of your control due to occupational practices

- What you do when you go out to eat or when eating at a party

YOUR PERSONAL EXERCISE FORMULA

Now that you have a working model for your diet formula, I want to briefly summarize a few details regarding your personal exercise formula. Remember, diet and exercise must work together to maintain a healthy metabolism and keep you on track to meet your weight-loss goals.

In chapter 5 I addressed various types of exercise styles that are beneficial to your health. When properly combined, you will be able to maximize your ability to achieve your exercise goals in the shortest period of time. In implementing your personal exercise formula, I suggest that you combine all the exercise styles for a set number of minutes each. Then progressively intensify the workout over a three- to four-month program. The amount of time you have reserved for exercise will remain the same; it will be the intensity of the routine that increases as you progress.

For those who really want to get the "ripped" beach body look, I invite you to visit my website at www.schoolofwellness.com and preview "The Gen-Intensity Workout." Otherwise, I recommend that you follow the exercise plan I have outlined in this text.

Consistency

The key to being successful with any exercise program is consistency. Sometimes we believe that joining a gym or buying a piece of exercise equipment or TV fitness program is the solution, but in reality they are just tools to create the success, not the driving force to initiate or sustain the success. Another fact I have learned, as both the doctor and the coach, is that everyone is different in their exercise ability, motivation, and preferences.

Some people find doing crunches and lunges first thing in the morning in a quiet room extremely boring, but doing a similar exercise on their computer-generated training game to be tons of fun. Others are just pragmatic. They do the exercises in the morning and then just check it off the list as done! The ideal approach is to find something you like to do or a way you like to do it; then do it. Regardless of your approach, the success formula remains the same: slow incremental changes, including additions to your exercise program, over a long period of time.

Implementing the plan

Plan to start slowly, only three minutes of exercise per day for the first week. Your goal is to get to twenty minutes of exercise per day within seven to eight weeks. After that, plan to intensify the twenty minutes of daily exercise every week for the next six months. You may be saying to yourself, "Three minutes a day, that's simple; I can do that with no problem." Sure you can, so let's start doing it, three minutes every day for seven days straight.

The fact is that about 50 percent of the patients who start my program in my office, even after paying cash, admit that after the first week they didn't do the three minutes of exercise every single day. So I have them start again, but with a sterner tone that lets them know, as their personal coach, I mean business. How can I expect them to be accountable for the larger tasks if they can't be accountable to this smaller task? Most of the time they get the idea by week two. The purpose for basing the formula on slow incremental changes over a long period of time is to develop permanent, new success-based habits. Own what you do, and you will do what you own.

Congratulations! With this information regarding your diet and exercise formulas in hand, you are ready to begin Week 1 of your personal wellness plan.

Chapter 7

THE GENESIS PROCESS (WEEK 1)

NOW WE'RE READY to begin the process of setting a plan to follow that will assure your success in reaching your wellness goals. Unlike many self-help, get-yourself-into-shape books, I am not a big fan of "spoon-feeding" my patients non-thought-provoking recipes or forcing them to follow a "my way or the highway" formula. Some weight-loss programs sound good, at least from a sales and marketing perspective, offering you a step-by-step, "you don't have to think" formula for getting into shape. But I like to see people take ownership of their fitness goals by using their creativity. Taking that responsibility means that when they reach their goals, they will not be as likely to quit the program and return to their unhealthy habits; they have established a healthy lifestyle for lasting results.

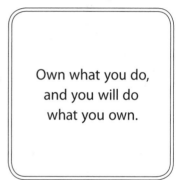

Own what you do, and you will do what you own.

As you know, our society has been gradually groomed to expect fast, easy results in many aspects of life. Because of our overwhelmingly busy lifestyles, anything that gives the impression it can minimize our physical and mental efforts is appreciated. It is still a fact, however, that every major achievement in life comes at the cost of the hard work of developing success attitudes that create success habits.

COACHING FOR PERSONAL SUCCESS

Please understand, I firmly believe in following an exact strategy for your personal health goals. The key word here is *personal*; one size does not fit all. Your personal health plan has to be built around your strengths, weaknesses, likes, and dislikes. Every great athlete, no matter their enormous talent, has to develop success-based habits for continuous physical training. Developing great success habits that feel natural to you and for which you can take ownership is the best methodology to achieving lasting results.

In my style of "doctoring," I consider myself more of a personal coach than a "sit-behind-the-desk" doctor. I believe a great coach works with the talent of his team to make them successful without trying to conform his players to his plan, making them become someone they are not. A great coach strives to recognize the talents, skills, and demeanor of his or her players. Then they work with their athletes' strong points to develop a winning team.

I believe that every patient has the ability to be successful in improving his or her health goals. Of course, I would never encourage someone to believe in a goal that, professionally, I do not think is possible. But after twenty-five years in practice, I have learned never to discourage anyone from believing because, as Jesus said, "with God all things are possible" (Matt. 19:26). I wrote the first chapters of this book to show you the importance of obedience to the Word of God, embracing His covenantal principles that promise health and well-being.

Now I would like to develop for you a working outline of how to get started in the first week of your Genesis Life Seven Weeks to Wellness program. The chart shows the health points that you will need to implement during the first week.

GENESIS LIFE HEALTH POINTS—FIRST WEEK

- The Food Diary Log
- Three minutes of abdominal exercises
- Addressing supplementation
- Assessing rest
- Assessing water
- Assessing stress levels and source
- Neurological assessment

IMPLEMENTING THE FOOD DIARY LOG

In chapter 5 we discussed in detail the purpose for and the way to use the Food Diary Log (FDL). As you begin the first week of your program, the purpose for completing the FDL is solely for getting yourself accustomed to recording everything you eat. It will also help you to recognize your present eating habits. You become aware of the times of day you eat, your food choices, the quantities of food you consume, and the various food groups you choose most often, as well as those you omit.

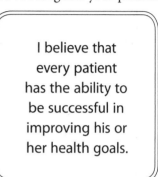

I believe that every patient has the ability to be successful in improving his or her health goals.

To begin, go to my website and print out the FDL. Then plan to begin tomorrow morning recording everything you eat and drink (other than water, which has a separate section). Remember to record the exact time you eat and the description of the food, including an accurate quantitative measurement of the portion. This process may seem tedious at first, but mastering these details will give you confidence and expertise to master the more challenging points later on.

You will probably notice at the end of this first week (like many of my patients) that you have some bizarre eating habits. From the information you have received in earlier chapters, you understand better what constitutes proper food choices and timing of meals. From your log, determine how many meals you skip, how much junk food you really eat, how much of a carboholic you are (extreme consumer of carbohydrates), and that you probably don't eat nearly the amount of vegetables you thought. If your FDL looks like a dietary disaster, don't fret. That's a good thing. It means you were honest and accurate; whatever you recorded was a great accomplishment.

The fact that you are writing down what you eat will subconsciously alter some of your eating habits almost automatically. That is especially true when you know you have to show your Food Diary Log on a weekly basis to someone to whom you are accountable. As we have discussed, *accountability* is the key to your ultimate success. Earlier when I addressed the need for accountability, I said that the ideal person to choose for accountability is someone who knows more than you and has a vested interest in your personal success. In case no one comes to mind, let me offer some possibilities:

- Move to New York City and make an appointment with me for Monday morning. I know, while this may be an effective solution, it will not always be practical.

- Find a doctor in your area on our website (www.schoolof wellness.com) who participates in the Genesis Diet program.

- Find a mentor on our website with whom you can buddy up. This trained person will serve as an accountability partner and source for encouragement and support.

- Get a friend to partner with you. Even if they don't fit the criterion of knowing more than you, they can be a source of accountability, especially if they're as serious as you are in your quest to get into great shape. Your best choice would be a good friend whom you know you can trust and has trusted you in the past with other life issues. Note: Sometimes spouses, siblings, parents, and children are not always the best choice. But I have seen it work, especially with some mother-daughter and father-son partners.

Whatever your solution, the accountability factor is essential for you to succeed with your FDL as well as your entire health protocol. Someone needs to look at your log with a critical eye, someone who can encourage you to make changes needed.

So what are we looking for on your FDL during the first week, and where do you begin to make changes? We discussed in chapter 6 the general purpose for each type of information you are recording. Now it is time to get more specific to help you enter the correct information into your FDL.

Evaluating the time column

Your main objective for timely eating during the day is to manage your food intake in intervals of two to two and a half hours, totaling six meals each day. Assuming that your busiest activity occurs during the middle of the day, the optimal goal for calorie intake is for your first and second meals to be smaller, increasing the amounts of food in your third and fourth meals, and decreasing amounts again for your last two meals toward the end of the day.

Referring to the sample FDL (Appendix A), you can see that your first meal should contain approximately 10 percent of your total projected calorie limit. Your second meal should be 15 percent, your third and fourth meals 25 percent each, and your fifth and sixth meals 15 percent and 10 percent respectively.

From this sample formula you should be able to modify this eating plan according to your personal daily activities, keeping the same pattern of eating larger quantities during the times of the day you are the busiest and have the greatest need for available energy.

At the beginning, for the sake of your training, it is more important to establish a habit of eating timely meals than it is to learn to manage caloric volumes. Once you develop and establish the habit of spreading out multiple meals properly throughout the day, you can focus in subsequent weeks on the caloric volume factor. Even if the caloric volumes of the meals don't match the sample FDL, the fact that your meals were spaced out properly during the day is a very good start. Eventually, by means of slow incremental changes, you will get to the goal of correct calorie intake in each food category as well.

As long as you progressively work toward the goal of consuming the correct percentage of calories that corresponds to your activity levels during the day, you will make progress. This timely eating pattern will keep you from dumping excess glucose into the bloodstream during an inactive time of the day, which inevitably leads to unwanted and unhealthy fat creation.

Recording your food breakdown column

The first task is just to get into the habit of accurately recording a quantitative amount and exact description of the foods. *Quantitative* means a measurable volume such as ounces and cups. Exact *description* means including terms like whole wheat, whole grain, fried, baked, steamed, and so on. The development of this habit is essential, especially when you begin to create alternative substitutions for common food sources.

As you get into the habit this first week of recording everything you eat, you can also be reviewing the Eat Sheet (see Appendix C), which gives you an idea of the caloric value of the foods you are eating. Many people notice after recording their meals that they are creatures of habit when it comes to the variety of foods they eat. The average person eats fifteen to twenty different meal combinations. For that reason, in a short period of time you will able to memorize the caloric values of your foods without referring to the Eat Sheet chart. If you eat foods that are not listed on that chart, just do an Internet search for the food to find its caloric value.

Goal for food category columns

Your goal by the end of the first week is to begin to record the caloric value for each food in its proper category. You want to learn to manage the quantity of calories allowed in each food group, without exceeding the desired target amount. Eventually you will learn to follow the increasing/decreasing pattern of consumption discussed earlier.

If you look at the sample FDL in Appendix A, the 2:00 p.m. meal shows 3 ounces of salmon, ½ cup of brown rice, and 2 cups of vegetables. The category columns show:

- 10 calopoints, or 100 calories, in the C (carbohydrate) column for the ½ cup of brown rice

- 12 calopoints, or 120 calories, in the P (protein) column for the salmon

- 6 calopoints, or 60 calories, in the V (vegetable) column for the vegetables

- 4 calopoints, or 40 calories, in the BO (butter/oils) column for the dressing or butter on the vegetables

The total calories for this meal are 320, which is approximately 25 percent of the total calorie target for the day. More importantly, the 10 points or 100 calories from the rice leaves a balance of 260 calories allowed for the carbohydrate column for the rest of the day. Using this precise, visual method of subtraction will help you manage each of the food groups throughout the day.

In essence, the FDL will guide you to manage several target numbers at the same time:

- Total number of calories for the day

- Total calories per each food group per day

- Total calories per meal as a percentage of the whole

Of the above-mentioned targets, the first and most important habit to develop is the tracking of the *total calories per each food group* per day. I suggested earlier that you treat each column as if it's a bank account, keeping in mind that each account has different guidelines and consequences for improper eating. For example:

- The *carbohydrate* column is an account with severe overdraft charges. Going over the limit means you are creating and storing fat.

- The protein account can also create problems when the limit is exceeded: increased acidity in body chemistry, decreased digestive function, and increased blood levels of cholesterol and triglycerides. Also, increased protein consumption without carbohydrates (high-protein diets) can produce weight loss, but usually at the risk of the above imbalances. In addition, they are rarely sustainable over a long period of time.

- The vegetable account, on the other hand, has reward points if you go over your number. Those rewards are called good health!

- The fruit account is best served if you stay at the target number. This is not to say that eating too much fruit can be unhealthy for you, but certain fruits are very high in sugars and have a glycemic index number that may be problematic. I mentioned pineapple with its powerful digestive enzymes. Though good for you, it is high in sugar and has a high glycemic index. In addition, I recommend that if you go over your limit in your fruit account, you add those additional calories to your carbohydrate account. This may not be an even exchange, but it is important that you hold all your accounts accountable!

- The dairy account is not an account of necessity, in my opinion. I created this account for those who feel they have to have their milk and cheese. It is not an account that you have to try to reach the maximum intake. If you score a zero at the end of the day, it's no big nutritional deal. On the other hand, going over the account limit does generate another source to promote fat production.

- The butter and oil account, much like the dairy account, is necessary to track your overuse of them; it is not a necessary target that you need to reach. There is no real reason to strive to consume foods that have points in this category. Butter, oils, and dressings that contain oils are mainly for seasoning, not nutritional enhancement. The health argument, of course, is for olive oil. It is true that "unheated" extra-virgin olive oil is high in unsaturated fats, which actually provides a health benefit to the cardiovascular system. The downside is that once the oil is heated for sautéing, it becomes denatured and loses its nutritional benefit; at 120 calories per tablespoon, it does no good for your overall calorie count.

BEGINNING YOUR THREE-MINUTES-A-DAY EXERCISE ROUTINE

This first week you need to begin taking my exercise challenge. I explained that the goal for this week is to perform three minutes of abdominal exercise each day for seven days. That's it. For those who routinely go to the gym, this goal may seem ridiculously easy. Conversely, there may be some people who aren't doing three minutes of exercise per year! The point is to begin making small incremental changes in your exercise habit for life.

With your three minutes of abdominal exercise, you will begin establishing a daily level of consistent exercise and accountability. Some avid gym goers will have a tough time meeting this challenge to complete this simple exercise routine *every* day for a week. Most people don't go to the gym every day. If you are in the habit of exercising at the gym only, there will be days you don't exercise at all. You will need to adjust to this seven-day routine to insure your success.

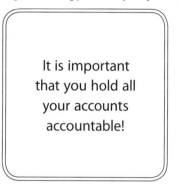

It is important that you hold all your accounts accountable!

The goal of the three-minute ab exercise, which will eventually develop into a twenty-minute full-body exercise routine, is to create a foundational standard of daily exercise, whether or not you go to the gym several times a week. Even if you do a thorough workout at the gym, I suggest that you make this in-home exercise routine part of your daily activity.

Instruction for your basic abdominal exercise

The basic abdominal exercise is called a crunch. Correct positioning for this exercise is essential to create maximum benefit and to decrease the chance of physical injury. You can view a video of the proper execution of this exercise on my website, www.schoolofwellness.com, in the free resources section.

Otherwise, you can begin your three-minute exercise by lying on your back on a firm but cushioned surface. In most cases a carpeted floor works, but if you need more cushioning, a mat or towel can be added for comfort. Your fluffy bed is not a recommended surface because it will alter the mechanics of the exercise; my real fear is that you may fall asleep before the three minutes are up!

Lying flat on your back, bend your knees comfortably so that the soles of your feet are flush on the ground. Interlock your hands and put them behind your neck (not your head). This will support your neck and decrease the chance of neck strain when performing the exercise. The exercise is simple, but I like to break it down into three steps:

1. First, gradually contract your lower abdominal muscles and tilt your pelvis upward. (Believe it or not, this is the most difficult part of the exercise.) If you are doing this correctly, you will notice that your buttocks will come slightly off the ground while the top of your sacrum (where your pelvis meets your spine) will become more flush against the floor. As you roll your pelvis upward, your abdominal muscles should be increasing their contraction and your entire lower spine should be getting flatter against the floor.

   At this point your upper back, neck, and head area should still be in contact with the floor. If you notice your entire buttocks coming off the floor, you have engaged your gluteal muscles, counteracting the contraction of the ab muscles. If you notice your belly area rising off the floor, you're probably engaging your lower back muscles, which will defeat the purpose of the exercise entirely. Sometimes it takes a while to coordinate the contraction and movement of the muscles.

2. The next step is to contract the upper part of the abdominal muscles by concentrating on bringing the lower edge of your rib cage toward your belt line while holding the pelvic contraction in step 1 in place. As your ribs contract toward your belt, your upper back will come off the ground, as well as your head and neck area. It is very important to have your hands behind your neck and focus your eyes upward. There is no need to look down toward your abs. Looking straight up as you go through the contraction will better support your head and cause less strain on your neck.

3. Once you master the mechanics for these two contractions (steps 1 and 2), you are ready to perform the exercise. The objective is to contract the abdominals from both directions and hold for six seconds. Then release, back to the floor in a resting posture.

The plan is to repeat this three-step crunch action for three minutes without stopping. From a repetition perspective, the goal would be to do ten crunches per minute, totally thirty at the end of the three minutes. For those who find this exercise difficult at the beginning, don't get discouraged. Remember, the overall priority is to become committed to setting aside the *time* allotted for exercise to help you toward your wellness goal.

For your encouragement, I don't care if you get on the floor and only accomplish three crunches in three minutes, as long as you honestly tried. If you really did give it your best effort, the next day you'll get to six crunches and eventually you'll get to the target number, even if it takes four weeks instead of one.

Never get discouraged because of lack of your present abilities. Who cares? You're doing this for you. It is not a race, and no one is judging you. As long as you're sticking to the plan and rebuking the excuses and negative chatter of the enemy to discourage you, you will eventually be successful.

These abdominal crunches are the starting place for your exercise plan. If this is simple to achieve, you can probably move on to the next exercise steps sooner. But for the first week, the bottom line is that you are committed to doing these abdominal exercises *every* day—not four out of seven days and not "most" of the time.

This beginning exercise routine is part of developing new habits. So, just because this is easy for you to do doesn't mean you have the option of missing one day, thinking you can make it up the next day or substitute going to the gym. The eventual habit of successfully developing your twenty-minute daily exercise routine begins with this three minutes of exercise a day—period.

ADDRESSING SUPPLEMENTATION

As you begin your first week of the program, you should also consider your need for *nutritional supplements* to replace nutrients that are absent from our best food sources. Even most family doctors now recommend a good multivitamin-mineral formula to their patients because of our deteriorating quality of food. Of course, all vitamins and minerals are not created equal. And there are no "perfect" pills to swallow for optimal health.

If you have ever watched a vitamin or nutritional supplement infomercial on television, you may have wondered if some of the unbelievable claims are actually true. Could it be that a pill has the power to block the fat from being absorbed in your intestine? Or a powder will really control your appetite? Or, my favorite, the supplement you swallow just gets the fat off your belly? How about the vitamin formula that is to end all other vitamin formulas? Or the herbal blend that claims to provide total physiological restoration without the need for diet, exercise, or neurological correction?

With the sudden public awareness of large-scale deficiencies of vitamin D in the population, supplement manufacturers, TV personalities, and well-known ministers are all cashing in on the fear factor created by the publicity. Sure, there is sound research to support the fact that vitamin D (along with many other nutritional factors) is necessary for the promotion of good health and to prevent cancer, heart disease, and many other chronic and debilitating diseases. But to create a paradigm for the public that says vitamin D is the latest "cure-all and prevent all" is ludicrous and borderline dangerous.

Here's the true test of a product's validity. How many of those supplements will still be on television five years from now? Also, did the product live up to the hype of the commercial? Does the product really look out for the overall health of the consumer? The answer to all those questions is *NO*.

How can I be so dogmatic? Because it is simply irresponsible to promote the idea that taking any single vitamin, herbal formula, or any other "so-called" natural concoction can replace all other factors involved in a person's quest for natural wellness. My philosophy is that supplements are designed to supplement what you may not regularly get in your normal diet. Their purpose is limited to promoting the well-being of various systems in the body.

Historical search for natural remedies

For thousands of years in many different cultures, people have, by trial and error, identified specific plant and herbal by-products that could make obvious physiological changes to the function and activity of particular organs and glands. Today, reputable research organizations have proven that there are exact compounds of these herbal extracts that can conclusively promote wellness, with little or no side effects.

As you know, your body is made up of many different organs and glands, which combine their efforts to function in various physiological systems.

Their sole purpose is to work in unity to promote the overall wellness of your body. When disease or illness strikes, it is natural to look for an external source to remedy the problem. With that in mind, let me share my thoughts on supplementation.

System support and prevention

Certain systems in the body are paramount to the function of other systems and, in turn, to the overall function of the entire body. Nutritional supplements that promote the well-being of these major systems—your cardiovascular system, immune system, digestive system, sugar metabolism, liver detoxification, and cleansing of the large intestine—are advisable for everyone, regardless of present complaints or lack of them. This school of thought is based on the idea of ongoing system support and prevention of disease, as opposed to a reaction to ailments that medicates with natural products in lieu of pharmaceuticals.

During my years of chiropractic practice, I have developed three herbal-vitamin-mineral formulas to address this issue of supporting these major physiological systems and biological functions. At no time will I ever claim that these are the best products in the world. And I will never mislead my patients to believe that taking these supplements alone is the remedy for all that ails them. That said, they have proved helpful to many, and, of course, I can vouch for their quality. If you are interested in evaluating these natural supplements, I invite you to go to www.schoolofwellness.com and click on the category: "What's in the supplements?"

Regardless of where you purchase your supplements, I firmly believe that, with few exceptions, you would benefit from system-supporting supplementation. The following chart can be a guideline for choosing quality supplements.

CONSIDERATIONS FOR SUPPLEMENTATION

> • Herbal preparations and combinations are a better choice than synthetically based vitamin formulas.

- Powdered formulas are usually better absorbed and have a higher level of bioavailability than solid tablets.

- It is better to purchase products on recommendation and research than by asking "What's the best price?"

- Be wary of products that are built into a multilevel marketing program—not because they are necessarily bad products (some can be excellent), but because they usually come with the most grandiose claims, they're usually very expensive, and a financial commission rather than your need usually motivates the sale.

- Focus on system-based supplementation like that previously mentioned. The only addition that may be needed is cod liver oil (yuck), which is a great source of (you guessed it) vitamin D and essential fatty acids.

Taking your supplements

Once you get your supplements, be sure to follow the recommendations for their use. More importantly, put them in an obvious place so that you are sure to take them. I know from experience with hundreds of patient confessions that regularly taking supplements can be a challenge for people, especially if they are not accustomed to taking any type of pills. They simply forget.

The objective is to establish a plan that increases your compliance. Here's my solution. Since most herbal formulas are considered a food, they can be taken without meals to assist their absorption. There is also little chance of upsetting the stomach. I keep my Detox and Antioxidant formula next to my bed with a bottle of water. When I wake up, I just pop two capsules with water and off I go. I keep my cod liver oil gels in an obvious place in the refrigerator (to avoid rancidity). So, when I go to the kitchen to make a little breakfast, the bottle is right there when I open the refrigerator door. Finally,

I have my Digestion formula sitting on my desk at the office. My largest meals are usually in the middle of the day. It is an easy habit to maintain to take one or two Digestion formula capsules after I finish eating.

Again, optimal wellness is all about creating habits that fit into your lifestyle. Figure out in advance how to strategically place your supplements in your home or office so that you are almost tripping over them. An additional help will be your Food Diary Log, where the last column is designated "S" for supplements; check off if you have taken your supplements. Remember, the tools are there to guide you until it all becomes a habit.

ASSESSING YOUR REST

Here's the simple question you need to answer: Do you get enough rest? In chapter 5 we discussed how getting adequate rest helps you avoid the unnecessary emotional stress associated with the lack of sleep. Sleep deprivation can go unrecognized for many years; you may just consider it a part of your "way too busy" lifestyle. The main physiological purpose for getting enough rest is simply to give the cells in your body time to recuperate from the activity of the day.

How do you know if you are getting enough rest? Here is my simple, nonclinical test to help you answer that question: When you have a day off or you are on vacation and there is no pressing reason to get up in the morning, how do you feel when you wake up? If you physically feel rested, calculate the number of hours you slept. That will give you a good idea of how many hours you need to sleep to get enough rest.

The only glitch is for those people with the built-in biological alarm clock (like me) that wakes you up early. If that happens, when you awaken, just lie there and relax, pray, fill your mind with pleasant thoughts, and don't get up until you absolutely can't lie there any longer. Then calculate the hours from when you went to bed until you got out of bed as the amount needed for optimal rest.

If you don't typically get the hours of sleep you calculated for feeling rested, try going to bed earlier. For example, perhaps you are in the habit of going to bed at midnight and have to wake up at six o'clock to get ready for work. Every day when you wake up, the first words you say are "I'm exhausted." You drag yourself around your room in denial, mumbling that you can't believe morning has come so fast. Reality would conclude that six hours may not be enough rest. If you tried my pseudoscientific sleep experiment, you may have realized that you need eight hours to truly wake up rested.

To wake up rested, you need to start implementing slowly a plan for sleep modification. The next night intentionally shut the TV off, get into bed, and close your eyes at 11:45 p.m. For the next seven nights, intentionally set your bedtime fifteen minutes earlier each night so that by the end of the week your new bedtime would be 10:00 p.m.

Somewhere in your sleep modification process, you will find a bedtime that will help you greet the morning with a smile instead of a frown. After increasing your sleeping time from six to eight hours a night, if you still feel exhausted on a workday, you might need to consider that the problem is not physiological. You may be suffering from a sleep disorder, which can be treated. Or maybe it's time to look for a new job!

Always remember, any changes you make should be incremental, as I described. Keep in mind, especially during the first week of your Genesis Diet program, you don't want to make too many shocking changes to your body.

Assessing Your Water Intake

Whenever I do my Wellness Workshop Presentation, I usually ask the audience to self-evaluate some of their regular wellness habits: How often do you eat whole grains? Do you exercise twenty minutes daily? Do you believe you get enough rest? Do you think you drink enough water every day?

I have observed that the water question gets the most favorable response. It almost seems that people think because they have bought into hydration, that makes up for all the other bad habits that plague their lifestyle. That said, it is important that during the first week of the program you keep track of the frequency and the amount of water you normally drink.

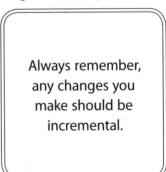

Always remember, any changes you make should be incremental.

The purpose for this assessment of your water intake is not so much to know the *amount* you drink but to make you aware of all your beverage choices. What do you choose to drink during the day? Why? For example, some people have to have coffee or tea in the morning to get them going. Some people need the flavor of juice or the fizz of soda, and others feel they must have milk on their cereal.

The point of tracking your water consumption is to help you develop the habit of drinking water as a practical first choice. Incorporating more water consumption can be done in simple ways. Your diet soda at lunch can easily be replaced by a bottle of water. Drink a large glass of water in the morning as a substitute for one of your cups of coffee.

On the other hand, though I'm not a big fan of dry cereal and milk, I wouldn't recommend that you put water on your cereal, since the very idea sounds gross. However, oatmeal and some other hot cereals have an alternative recipe that uses water instead of milk, a healthier choice in my opinion.

Water should be your drink of choice whenever you have the slightest sense of thirst. It is not a bad idea to carry a water bottle with you at all times. In addition, raw vegetables and fruits are naturally high in purified water as well as essential vitamins and minerals.

For the first week your task is to simply track your normal water consumption on your FDL. Also make a note of all the times you drank a beverage other than water. This will give you a good idea of whether or not you are truly drinking enough water and make you aware of times water would have been a better choice. I have observed that it is rare that people drink too much water; it is very easy to not drink enough.

ASSESSING YOUR DAILY STRESS LEVELS

It is always easier said than done when it comes to reducing our stress levels. Whenever we see a friend who is stressed out, our natural instinct is to give them advice on relaxing, suggesting that they take a deep breath and think the matter through before taking any action. Often our friends do the same for us when we are stressed, expressing their concern. The problem with a sympathetic pat on the back or advice regarding what you *should* have done is that it offers no real solution to your excessive stress level.

The main consequence of living with stress is, of course, the unhealthy physiological changes it causes in your body. As I discussed earlier, emotional stress creates a hyperactive function of your organs and glands, eventually leading to serious malfunction and chemical toxicity. So how do we eliminate the inevitable?

Handling self-induced stress

In our earlier discussion regarding the effects of stress on your health, we concluded that you must try to identify and minimize the stress in your life. Certain stress situations are unavoidable and inescapable just because we are humans and we live in a world that is far from perfect. But it is also true that a certain percentage of our stress is self-induced. Here is where we need to do an honest and transparent self-evaluation of certain aspects of our lives, which become typical playgrounds where stressful events occur.

Once you are able to identify the stress that originates, at least in part, in your personal decisions, choices, or actions, you will be able to make definite choices to bring resolution to your stress. How can you be sure which stressful situations are self-created? How can you be sure that the actions you will take will actually bring resolution to the stress?

Of course, the answer to those questions is not cut and dry. And I am not a psychiatrist with the perfect answer. However, as a student of the Word of God, I can tell you that any of our actions or decisions that are contrary to the Word of God will always result in chaos and stress. The prudent person who wants to resolve self-induced stress levels will need to assess their actions, words, and decisions in light of biblical principles we discussed earlier. Unfortunately, even many believers are deficient in their knowledge of God's covenantal provisions and promises, as well as the consequences for violating them, that govern the outcome of all our actions.

So where do you start? First, you need to accept the fact that being "stressed out" *will always be a hindrance* in your quest for getting into shape. Second, be honest and work to address the obvious areas that are causing the most stress. This means owning up especially to areas of your lifestyle where you have broken covenant.

Earlier we discussed that covenant means a pact or an agreement that God makes with His people in order to bless them, preserve them, and prosper them. Every instruction God gave mankind in His Word was to assure their well-being and to give them dominion over every creature in this world. In Genesis 1:26 when God said, "Let Us make man in Our image, according to Our likeness," He also covenanted to give them dominion over everything in the earth.

Remember, a covenant is a binding contract, whether or not a person decides to embrace its requirements. When God decided to make mankind, He set into motion the requirements of divine covenant that would assure those who obeyed them good success in every area of life. The converse is also true; covenant breakers will suffer consequences for not walking in obedience to these biblical principles.

Where stress is concerned, violating God's principles regarding relationships, finances, forgiveness, or any other aspect of life results in self-induced stress levels that can wreck your health. I have observed the following life involvements that seem always to be at the base of stressful situations:

- Stress in the marriage relationship

- Stress in the parent/child relationship

- Stress in the child/parent relationship

- Stress in the job situation

- Stress in the area of finances

- Stress in the area of health

In chapter 10 I will address each of these areas in greater detail, but your assignment for the first week is to simply *write down*, in detail, the problems you may be having in any of the above-mentioned areas of your life, or others of which you are aware. It is critical to develop awareness of what's stressing you out in order to learn where you need to search for solutions to your self-created stress. Owning your stress, instead of blaming the other person or situation, is important to resolving it.

YOUR NEUROLOGICAL ASSESSMENT

At first glance, you may think that your neurological assessment has to do with the state of your mental health. It does not. Rather, it applies to the *anatomical and physiological function* of the nervous system itself. This is not as complicated as it sounds. *Anatomical* function deals with the actual *physical structure* of the nervous system, which includes the brain, spinal cord, and the spinal nerves. *Physiological* function deals with the *actual operation* of the nervous system, which includes the transmission of neurological signals from the brain, through the nerves, to every part of the body.

The premise for living a healthy life is to understand that the brain controls all the functions of the body. Therefore, a properly functioning nervous system allows all the muscles, organs, and glands of the body to function at 100 percent. Without proper neurological communication from your brain to your stomach, it would be impossible for your stomach to function normally. That is true for any organ in your body; the root cause of your physical distress could be a dysfunction in your neurological system.

I have observed that most people with stomach disorders, for example, never consider neurological interference as a possible cause of their condition. Most assume that the cause is dietary or stress-related and proceed to take medications to treat the stomach's symptoms and make them "feel better." Some people make wise decisions to correct their diet and take measures to reduce their stress rather than popping pills for relief.

These lifestyle changes will definitely help. But if the problem persists, it is time to check the "controlling power," your brain, to see if there is a neurological malfunction that needs to be investigated. This hypothesis is valid for every system in the human body. It just makes sense that if the communication from the brain to the body is impeded, that system affected would fail to function at its maximum potential.

How it works

Now that we understand the importance of proper neurological communication for health, let's examine possibilities of physical interference. The neurological signal generated by the brain is in the form of an electrochemical impulse. It travels almost at the same speed as an electrical current does through the wire of your telephone. Like your telephone, the quality of the signal depends on the clear passage of the transmission from its source to the receiver. Any interference will alter the flow of the signal, causing a garbled or static-filled reception.

Now picture this happening in your body. Your brain is in constant communication to every part of your body, and the slightest interference in neurological transmission can lead to a system breakdown. I will discuss more specifically later how the nervous system can impact your overall health. For now, let me strongly suggest that you set up a consultation with your family chiropractor who can give you a spinal checkup to detect any potential nerve interference in any area of your body.

Let me reiterate that my main concern is your *overall wellness*. Losing weight and building muscle mass just for the sake of satisfying your vanity will serve no lasting purpose; it will only make you look good while you are getting sick. I encourage you to mark this page and refer to the Quick Review chart often to make sure you are completing everything assigned for your first week of the program.

QUICK REVIEW: WEEK 1

- **The Food Diary Log**: Make sure you write down everything you eat and drink, paying special attention to the description and quantitative amount.

- **Three minutes of abdominal exercises:** This has to be done every day. My suggestion is to not leave your bedroom in the morning until these exercises are done. There is no use moving to more exercises unless you are accountable to these three initial minutes.

- **Addressing supplementation:** Check out the supplements on the www.schoolofwellness .com site or visit your local health food store and research similar products.

- **Assessing rest:** Follow the exercise in the chapter. The faster you determine the correct amount of time you need to rest, the better your overall outlook will be.

- **Assessing water intake:** Simply always have a water bottle at your disposal. When you are thirsty, choose to drink water!

- **Assessing stress levels:** Do the stress assessment and write it down. You can't correct something you're not sure you have control over.

- **Neurological assessment:** The proper transmission of neurological signals from your brain to your body is vital to the achievement of optimal health. Schedule an appointment with your family chiropractor. Go to my website at www.schoolofwellness .com to find possible information on locating a Genesis Diet program chiropractor in your area.

You are now armed with the tools needed for beginning the first week of the rest of your life. This first week of your program will set the stage for the rest of your efforts to achieve your health goals. Be committed to following the above steps precisely. As you have learned, this program advocates achieving your optimal health goals through small, slow incremental changes over a long period of time. That is why it works *for life.*

This methodology for wellness has been successful for many people who diligently follow it, helping them develop a lifestyle of wellness in every aspect of their lives. The final chapters will give you specific information for reaching your seven-week program to get into shape—for life.

As we discuss specifics of dietary substitutions, your personal exercise program, and how to deal with stress, you will be armed to complete the program and learn to develop a style of living to assure your optimal health. I will discuss the same topics we presented in earlier chapters, giving real-life examples, positive and negative, and specific instructions for each area of your health plan. My goal is to increase your understanding and motivate you to a firm commitment to living a life of wellness.

Chapter 8

TAKING DOMINION OVER YOUR DIET

M ANY YEARS AGO I had a baseball coach tell me that 90 percent of the game is won by just showing up mentally to play. The same is true for doing the Genesis Diet program or any other fitness/ weight-loss program in which you participate. My hope is that if you're reading this chapter, it's because you committed to starting this health program after reading the previous chapter. The purpose of this chapter is to give you further instruction to fine-tune the process that will optimize your chances of success.

You have shown your determination by reading the previous chapters and committing to begin Week 1 of the process. In doing so, you have applied Success Attitude #2: Take initiative. Getting the ball rolling is sometimes the hardest thing to do. Now, it is up to you to keep the ball rolling and to ramp up the momentum. So let's get you going on the road to success.

ESTABLISHING YOUR ACCOUNTABILITY

In chapter 3 I discussed the eight success attitudes, each of which is a covenantal principle to achieving optimal wellness. My experience has been that most of my successful patients have cultivated these dynamic traits in their pursuit of their health goals. And, as I have stated, it is my experience that the most influential success attitude for their long-term success was their willingness to be *accountable* to someone else who had more knowledge than they and a vested interest in them getting well.

Ideally, this accountability relationship occurs when you are my patient or another doctor's participating in our Genesis Diet program. What do you do if you're not? As I mentioned, the key here is to partner with people who will enhance your journey toward health, not be a hindrance. Never attempt to partner with someone who will be totally dependent on you for their own motivation or expertise.

Recently I had a group of three schoolteachers join the program in consultation with me at my office. Obviously, they would be accountable to me. But I also set up a situation where they would be accountable to one another. I told them that the three major areas of accountability are diet management, exercise compliance, and dealing with stress.

As it turned out, one of the teachers was very disciplined with shopping for food to prepare and organize a healthy food plan for the day. Another woman, who was a former athlete, was disciplined with doing daily exercises but had trouble managing her dietary habits. The last woman was admittedly neglectful when it came to diet and exercise, but being the school counselor, she helped her two friends deal with the stress of daily living.

This is an example of developing trust and accountability that are mutually helpful to the success of each person. Remember, the point of having someone partner with you is mainly for the object of accountability, not just to be a companion.

Making Real Adjustments in Your Diet

The goal for recording what you ate in the FDL in Week 1 was mainly to learn how to get into the habit of accurately writing down everything you eat. For some people this is a major challenge. In reality, it is one of the simplest forms of personal discipline. I have talked with thousands of unsuccessful dieters who admit that their biggest problem is a lack of discipline.

You don't have to be a nuclear physicist to understand that if it's discipline you lack, then it's discipline you need. Once you complete the first week of recording and observing the foods you ate, the quantities, and the time of day you ate them, it's time to start studying the results.

As you do, it should become obvious to you what your good and bad eating habits are. During the second week, your goal is to record the caloric value of the foods (calopoints) in the columns to the right in the FDL. Calculating these numbers will make it even more clear to you which eating habits need adjusting. (Please see Appendix C for my Eat Sheet; you may also access it on the free Genesis Diet page at www.schoolofwellness.com.) This Eat Sheet, as I mentioned earlier, is a basic guide to the approximate calories of foods in the various categories. You will notice that the calories are calculated into what I call "calopoints," dropping the last zero to make your addition easier.

During this second week, as you record calopoints for all foods you eat, you are also recording the time, description, and the amount of food. You will begin to memorize the caloric value of the foods you eat the most. Also, during the second week I want you to review the foods you ate in the first week. Go back and start adding in the calopoints and tabulate the numbers for each day. You will learn which categories you went over the target number and which ones you fell short of your target.

Also, you will notice which times of the day you skipped a meal or had a large gap of time between your meals. More than likely, if you felt the need for this program, you will notice that you usually went over your target amount in the carbohydrate section and were severely short in the vegetable column. And you probably had a gap of four hours or more at least once a day between meals. Whatever the outcome of your analysis of that first week, now is the time to start making adjustments.

The bucket rule

Earlier I discussed the importance of timely eating that does not shock your metabolism. When you space out your caloric intake to include six small meals at intervals of between two and two and a half hours, your sugar levels remain constant, which also promotes steady energy.

From a fitness and sugar metabolism perspective, it suits your body well to have a steady intake of small amounts of food rather than eating several huge meals spaced hours apart. People who load up on half their daily caloric intake at one time sometimes have a problem with planning meals. They may be involved in an occupation that prevents them from taking the time to eat smaller meals more often. Usually their concept of what prevents them from eating more often is based on a subjective perception of their current situation.

For example, you may think because you're a student, teacher, cashier, or any other kind of employee, you do not have the option of eating frequent meals. But that is simply not so. There is a way to get it done if you just learn to get creative. Remember, you have to think outside the box and do something different if you expect to get a different result.

The easiest solution to spread out your meals in a timely way is what I call the "bucket rule." When my daughter, Julie, was in high school, she was determined to follow my program and get into great shape. Like most students, she was faced with the predicament of how to spread out smaller meals appropriately, having to attend classes from 8:00 a.m. to 2:00 p.m. without a break. Instead of looking at a situation from a "what you don't have" perspective, it is important to consider the "what you do have" perspective.

Julie definitely didn't have time to sit down and have what we traditionally would consider a meal, but she did have short five- to seven-minute breaks between classes during which she could have a quick snack. She had to be creative and look at the seven short breaks between classes as one thirty-five- to forty-minute opportunity to eat.

As Julie prepared her meals for the next day, she would fill an 8-cup plastic container with about 700 calories of food, enough to sustain her energy level throughout the day. The bulk of the container she filled with spinach salad along with some grilled chicken or turkey slices, some goat cheese, some other raw vegetables, crushed almonds, and a few raisins.

Every day I would watch her preparing her container of food, wondering what she was doing. Not all teenagers are known for their organizational skills, and I thought it odd that she was so dedicated to this daily task. So I asked her, "What in the world are you doing with that food?" Her reply, in a typical "It should be obvious, Dad" tone was, "I'm filling my bucket of food for the day." So I said to myself, "Hmm…what a novel concept."

"Filling a bucket?" I asked. She then explained to me, the doctor, the simplicity of the concept. "Every day I fill this bucket with about 700 calories of food. In between classes I have a few minutes before the next class starts, so I open the bucket and pick out a little of the food. By the time I get home I have about three-fourths of the bucket eaten, which I eventually finish by 4:00 p.m." She concluded, "I'm never hungry during the day, and I'm never starving for a large dinner in the evening."

Julie went on to say that since she's been doing the bucket rule, she rarely reaches her calorie target and that she consistently reaches her vegetable goal for the day. She did get into shape, losing body fat, increasing muscle mass, and never feeling fatigued. In the following scenarios, you will see that the bucket rule could come in quite handy.

"Skip" a large meal late in the day.

Eating a large meal too late in the day is a problem for many people, especially for those of you who have three or four nights a week that you come home late from work. You have a typically long stressful day in which you had no time for lunch, and the day went on forever. When you finally get home, you're starving and you just want to eat.

I find that men confront this issue more than woman. Women who have a long stressful day tend to want to just collapse and go to bed. Men, on the other hand, usually have the desire to woof down a big meal, almost as if they deserved it because of the long and trying day they had. Then they collapse in front of the TV to catch the news or the scores of the games they missed. After their meal, they can't go to bed even if they wanted to because they're too full from the pound of pasta they just ate. You may be wondering why I chose pasta for this example and not a Caesar salad. The answer is that after long stressful day, you most likely crave a comfort food experience. Now, not only are you eating a meal late, you are also eating a large quantity of a type of food that may take forever to digest.

The physiological problem is obvious. A 500- to 800-calorie meal at the end of the day, when your activity level is least and will diminish even more when you go to bed, is a perfect scenario for your body to store fat. Within an hour after the meal, the blood sugar levels will begin to rise. By this time you're either zoned out in front of the TV or "out like a light" in bed. Your body has no other choice but to store most of the food you just ate as fat.

The matter is more complicated because you probably didn't spread out your earlier eating times, which created a large gap before you ate the large meal at night. As we discussed, this time lapse between meals will typically slow down your metabolism, creating an even greater opportunity to stress out your glandular system and store more fat when you do eat.

The obvious and probably the simplest solution would be to apply the bucket rule. If you know you're going to work late, create a bucket in the morning. If you don't expect to work late, but it just so happens that you do, then find a restaurant that can create a bucket for you. Take a few minutes to pick it up or get it delivered. This time dilemma is an opportunity to become proactive, not a time for excuses. It is easy to complain about the situation and somehow justify the big meal at 10:00 p.m., but what does that do for you from a health perspective?

I remember talking to a patient who had a huge problem trying to get over the late-night meal. Every week he would make his appointments and show sincere intent to get into shape. He lost a little weight (not nearly the amount the average overweight male should lose in the first few weeks of the program) and appeared to be diligent with his exercises. But he couldn't get the late-night meals under control.

Every week I would address the situation, and every week his response to me was an excuse. "Doc, you don't understand…" Eventually I would say, "You're right, I don't understand." And then one day, when his results were lagging and he made the same excuse, I said to him, "By the way, how's this working out for you?" He looked at me kind of confused and said, "What, the program?" "No," I said, "your excuses."

It took him awhile, but he finally realized that he was so accustomed to making the same excuse he actually began to believe it. The end of the story is that he took ownership for his eating situation. He found a diner that made a chicken salad, which was the perfect bucket-like solution for his late-night meal addiction.

Over on carbohydrates, short on vegetables

This high-carb/low-veggie scenario is by far the most common of FDL shortfalls. I still smile when I see the shock on my patients' faces when they see from their FDL how many carbs they eat and how few vegetables are actually on their daily menu. In reality it's very predictable for me.

For example, I interview a patient with the typical concern of finally making a decision to get into shape. Upon visual observation I can tell they are fifty pounds or more overweight, and the only gym they know is the "Jim" who works at the local deli. In a brief introduction of the program I always touch on the subject of lowering carbs and increasing vegetables. Then I wait to hear the classic line, "I love vegetables. I have no problem eating vegetables." Or this one, " I eat tons of vegetables." Clearly they must think I have a vision problem. My enthusiastic response to their skewed perception is always, "That's great."

What makes their "ton of veggies" comment more peculiar is when I ask them about eating carbs, and they tell me, "Oh, no, I'm not a big bread eater." Or they say, "I don't care for sweets." Later in the consultation, when I determine their body fat percentage is 50 percent and their BMR is close to 3,000 calories per day, often the truth starts dawning on them. "Well you know, Dr. V, I really love my ice cream." Or they say, "I am addicted to soda." Somehow we always get to the bottom of how to account for the 3,000 calories per day they are consuming.

The confirmation of their faulty eating habits always occurs in the first two weeks of the FDL review. The goal was to have 360 calories or less of carbohydrates and over 100 calories a day from vegetables. As I calculate the numbers, a consistent pattern emerges. Every day they are way over on the carbs, and even though they declared they "love vegetables," they are well below the target number for veggies. In many cases these people go two or three days (according to their FDL) without eating any greens at all.

Their original shock at the numbers brings them a good dose of reality for why they are in the shape they are. This reality therapy is the reason it is so important to write everything down. People honestly believe that they are not eating a lot of carbs and that they are getting plenty of vegetables.

How to fix the problem

Patty's story is helpful for learning how to eat less carbs and more vegetables. For her carbohydrate intake, she would have 1 cup of oatmeal in the morning, with a teaspoon of sugar and some raisins. Then she ate a turkey sandwich for lunch. In the late afternoon she would snack on "just a few" crackers and only eat ½ cup of brown rice with dinner. And while the rest of the family was eating pie and ice cream for dessert, she dutifully munched on two cookies.

In Patty's mind, she was cutting back on carbs and making some healthy eating choices. In reality, because she never ever recorded her food intake or added up the calories, she did not realize that her carb intake was out of line. When we took the calculator to the FDL, we noticed that Patty was 300 calories over her carbohydrate target for the day. Even if she kept the rest of her calories down in the other categories, she would still have trouble losing weight because she was putting her metabolism in fat storage mode. In addition, she was taxing the activity of the pancreas, adrenal glands, and digestive and immune systems, and she was continuously creating an acidic environment in the bloodstream. To make matters worse, Patty was one of the professed "vegetable lovers" who somehow had trouble recording even getting one serving of vegetables per day.

Using your FDL to help lower carbs and increase veggies

Here's where the FDL becomes an important tool. Patty's oatmeal was 160 calories, the bread from the sandwich was 240 calories, the crackers were 80 calories, the rice was another 100 calories, and finally the two cookies were 80 calories. How do we eliminate 300 of these carb calories? Let's start with the oatmeal. The oatmeal on its own is 120 calories, but the sugar and the raisins boost it up to 160 calories. To lower the carb count, you have to give up taste or give up volume. If you really need taste, then eat ½ cup and then have some fruit an hour later if you're still hungry. If you can manage around the taste, then just have the oatmeal plain. Either way you just saved 40 calories in your carb account.

Next is the turkey sandwich. Here you also have a few choices. One, you can have the turkey on an open-face sandwich (one slice of bread), put some extra lettuce and tomato on it, and eat it with a knife and fork, like an aristocrat. Or you can go Asian and eat it without bread, wrapping the turkey in large romaine lettuce leaves. In this case you can cut 120 to 240 calories off the carb account. If you eliminate the sandwich carbs altogether, you have reduced your carbs by 280 from the 300 you need to eliminate. If you went with the open-face sandwich (240 calories), the cookies for dessert that night are out of the question.

If you eliminate the crackers for a snack and substitute them with raw carrots, cucumbers, or broccoli, you're now at 360 reduced carbs. You could actually have more rice with the later meal.

Another good suggestion would be to intentionally "greenify" your starches (I just made up that word). It is possible to lower the volume of your pasta and rice intake by mixing green vegetables into the starch. For example, if you really love your rice and two of your favorite vegetables are spinach and peas, you could mix your spinach, peas, and rice together. The objective is to intentionally mix the greens with the starch to such a degree that you plate looks more green than white; hence, "greenified."

In this way you can eliminate some of the volume (calories) of the rice while still satisfying your desire for its taste and texture. Also, this is a great way to intentionally increase volume to the vegetable column on the FDL. Consider the impact on your calorie math. Normally you would have a 1½ cups of pasta in a serving with a cup of broccoli on the side. The pasta calories equal to about 300 and the broccoli maybe 20 calories.

The final calorie count comes out to about 320; the total volume of food is 2 ½ cups.

Now let's try to reduce some calories by "greenifying" the plate. Instead of 1 ½ cups of pasta, use only ¾ cup. Instead of 1 cup of broccoli, increase it to 2 ½ cups. The much greener plate is larger by ¾ cup volume. Yet it is 120 calories less than the original dish. The pasta at ¾ cup is now 150 calories, and the broccoli at 2 ½ cups is only 50 calories. You are eating more volume, getting more veggies, at significantly less calories.

This greenifying can be done with any combination of starch (rice, grains, pastas, potatoes, etc.) simply by mixing them with an increased amount of your favorite vegetables.

Short on vegetables—all the time?

Some people just don't eat vegetables. When they do, their concept of vegetables is corn and potatoes. Obviously you need to eat vegetables for their nutritional value to maintain optimal health. But more importantly, for the person who has to drop 100 pounds, there is a desperate need during the wellness program to create food volume by substituting low-calorie veggies for high-calorie foods.

I have seen hundreds of patients who fit this "no veggies" scenario. They love their carbs and proteins and are perplexed when I tell them that their favorite french fries are not in the vegetable family. A person who is fifty to one hundred pounds overweight usually has a BMR (daily calorie consumption rate) that is 2 to 2.5 times higher than needed.

What that means in real numbers is that in order for Big Joe to lose weight, he would have to lower his 4,500-calories-a-day diet to less than 2,000 calories a day. If he doesn't eat vegetables, this feat can be nearly impossible at first glance. In this situation we have to resort to the major mantra of this book: *slow incremental changes over a long period of time.*

Some patients, during the first two or three weeks of the program, look flustered when I point out to them another week has gone by and they have logged hardly any vegetables on their FDL. They always counter me with something like, "Doc, you need to look closer at my FDL. I put lettuce on my open-face sandwich, and I took your advice to mix my rice with peas." Sadly, these people are really trying. For them, a few leaves of lettuce and a couple of spoons of peas is a major accomplishment—not to mention that when they get on the scale, they have lost a few pounds. Small incremental changes are working.

If you are a no-veggies person, don't get flustered. Realize that making this change is just another step in the slow incremental changes on your road to success. Then make it a goal to consistently get more vegetables into your daily diet. The first step is to identify what vegetables you like and what vegetables you can at least tolerate. This is a key to your success, especially if your list is narrowed down to carrots only. In that case, you need to choose to be really open-minded. You have to have at least one or two types of leafy green (salad family) vegetables in your "like" or "tolerate" list. They are the essential ingredient for creating your daily bucket. That's right, we are revisiting the bucket concept.

Making a veggie plan

To go from no veggies to a reasonable daily intake of vegetables will require commitment to your health goals and a slow incremental plan. Let's say that your vegetable target is 120 calories per day, but your current vegetable consumption, recorded the first week, is only 20 calories per day (maybe you have 1 cup of broccoli with dinner). How can you increase that number? Here's where the bucket concept comes in handy.

As you begin the next week adjusting your food intake, determine to get your vegetable number up to 40 calories. To do that, you could fill your bucket with 1 cup of broccoli and 2 cups of romaine lettuce. The goal then is during your two biggest midday meals to make sure that you eat everything in the bucket that day. Once this becomes a consistent habit, increase the vegetable volume of the bucket to 60 calories. If you can add more and more each week to the bucket, by the end of a month or two you will automatically reach your target goal.

You will also notice, as you become more accustomed to eating vegetables from your bucket, that it is not difficult to prepare vegetables in a "normal" manner as a matter of course during your daily food preparation (for example, a fresh garden salad). That doesn't mean you should get rid of your daily bucket. If you're a busy on-the-go person, the bucket concept can be the perfect solution for your daily meal schedule.

Eating Correctly in a Typical Day

After you have identified your incorrect eating pattern, seeing trends logged in your FDL, begin to chart a plan for readjusting your eating schedule. A typical day might be that you wake up; grab a quick oatmeal, yogurt, or piece of fruit; and head out to work with your preprepared food bucket, filled the night before with the right combination of carbohydrates, vegetables, and proteins to carry you through the end of the day.

Always remember, your ultimate success depends on taking ownership of your new eating habits, designed by you. I am giving you ideas and healthy instructions, but in order to achieve a long-standing successful transition from bad habits to good habits, you must take ownership of the changes you make.

Receiving divine help

Looking to God for help to keep His covenant promises for health will also aid your success. I have mentioned that when God created mankind, He gave him dominion over the earth (Gen. 1:26, 28). That divine directive was intended for man's success, happiness, and total well-being. Then God said:

> Behold, I have given you every plant yielding seed that is on the surface of all the earth, and every tree which has fruit yielding seed; it shall be food for you.
>
> —Genesis 1:29

All seed-bearing herbs, plants, and fruits were designated to be consumed for our nutritional sustenance; they were the original food source, which became the foundation for building and strengthening our physical body. Seed-bearing vegetation also includes grains, beans, nuts, and fruits. So cheer up; you don't have to limit your food sources to broccoli or romaine. God was not narrow-minded in developing a menu for mankind.

Clearly, if you have a problem eating vegetables, it is not because God did not intend for you to eat them. He created your body to digest and process, and *enjoy*, seed-bearing vegetation. Please know that your present aversion to vegetables is a taste and texture issue, not a physiological mishap.

While I am not exclusively promoting a total vegetarian diet, I want you to understand the importance to your health, as God designed you, to feed your body an abundant variety of vegetables. They were the menu for Adam and Eve in the Garden of Eden. We can assume they were satisfying and health-giving to His first man and woman, as they should be for us.

How to reduce your protein count—and *why*

Eating too much protein is not as common as going over on the carbohydrates, but because it has its own pitfalls, it needs to be addressed. The high-protein diet became very popular in the 1990s as a trendy way to lose weight. The principle behind the practice was to basically eliminate carbohydrates from the diet and use protein sources as a primary food supply. From a weight-loss perspective, it proved to be rather favorable, at least for the short term.

The increase in protein along with the elimination of carbs creates a metabolic scenario in the body that uses fat to produce blood glucose for energy. This process is called putting the body into an unhealthy state of ketosis. While burning protein as your energy does work for weight loss, the nutritional backlash can become very problematic.

The increased protein consumption is usually accompanied with increased fat consumption. Protein sources from animal meats usually are very high in saturated fats, which are notorious agents for the propagation of heart disease, strokes, cancers, gout, and many other health conditions—not to mention that a high-protein/fat diet leads to a very acidic body chemistry, which again sets the stage for the proliferation of many health conditions, including autoimmune diseases.

The same way some people are hooked on carbs, others are hooked on protein. When they try eating a balanced diet, as my program proposes, their protein numbers can accumulate even faster than carb numbers because of their density and natural fat content. Linda's story can help you understand where you are regarding protein consumption levels.

Craving those proteins

Linda had no idea that she loved proteins so much. The first couple of weeks she filled out her FDL, she couldn't believe that she always went over her protein numbers. The rest of the categories seemed to be under control, but the proteins just keep on adding up even when she thought she was cutting back. A look at her daily diet told the story.

On a typical day Linda cooked scrambled eggs with cheese and two slices of bacon for breakfast. This calorie count would be 200 calories for the eggs, 100 calories for the cheese, and 90 calories for the bacon. Without counting the cheese, which can be part of the dairy count, her total was almost 300 calories. Her target for protein is 360 calories for the entire day. Not much left over for the rest of the day.

So she decided to modify the meal by using egg whites only and eating turkey bacon instead of pork bacon. This helped, but not as much as she thought. The egg whites were about 120 calories, and the turkey bacon was still about 75 calories, making her new breakfast protein number 195 calories. That is still kind of high for people who love their proteins throughout the day. Eating a grilled chicken cutlet for lunch or dinner would make her reach her target number for protein, with nothing to spare.

The proteins Linda ate are the lightweights of the category; beef, pork, and lamb carry some hefty caloric counts for very small portions. For example, a 6-ounce T-bone steak is about 340 calories, and a 4-ounce pork chop is about 260. As you can see, some protein sources have lots of calories that can really add up fast. So what can be done?

"I love meat."

If you are having trouble going over your protein target with meats, here are two options that will help you out. First, actively pursue *substitution*, and second, *create volume by chopping up the meats*. For example, it is fairly common knowledge that chicken, turkey, and fish are a healthier choice of protein than beef and pork, for several reasons. The fat content of the chicken, turkey, and fish is much less than the beef and pork. And some fish have the added benefit of high essential fatty acids, which actually promote a healthier cardiovascular, immune, and skeletal system.

From a strictly calorie-count aspect, consider that 4 ounces of grilled chicken is about 100 calories less than 4 ounces of a grilled pork chop, and 4 ounces of baked tilapia (fish) is 50 calories less than the grilled chicken. What it comes down to is simply learning to manage your protein calories based on the amount of volume of meat you desire to eat. For example, you can have two large baked flounder filets for less calories than one small lamb chop, with probably half the fat. By substituting the lower-fat, lower-calorie fish for other proteins, you can still eat meat and safely manage your FDL protein category.

What do you do if you are someone who hates fish? Obviously, the above factual explanation of the benefits of eating fish is not going to turn you into a fish-loving fisherman. So what option is there for those who are "real" meat eaters? The answer is to eat *less* meat by creating the illusion of volume. You can help to lessen your craving for meat by making it seem like you are eating more. This can be done effectively through the simple practice of chopping it up.

If you have ever ordered a salad with grilled chicken, you will know what I'm talking about. Some restaurants serve the dish with a whole grilled chicken cutlet sitting on top of the salad, while others serve the chicken as tenderloins. All you are thinking is, "I want a piece of chicken in every forkful of the salad."

By cutting the chicken, or any meat, into smaller than your usual (bite-size) pieces, you create the illusion of eating a greater volume of meat. Never mind that in reality you are just increasing the number of times you put meat into your mouth. Your craving for meat will be satisfied because your body "thinks" it ate a large volume, which was really just a larger number of mouthfuls.

As a side note, this chopping-up technique to create an illusion of volume also works for desserts and snacks. My wife can make one cookie last ten minutes by breaking it into small pieces and savoring the taste of each little bite as if it was an entire cookie. If you love cookies as much as some people love steak, you should do the same.

Addressing the egg question

There are a few ways to still have your eggs, deriving their best nutritional value, without piling up the calories. Lowering intake from two eggs to one is a big improvement for the calorie target, but it creates a void in the "what's on the plate" department. So, let's address this volume issue. We can use the same idea we did with carbs, adding vegetables to our egg dish to regain the volume. Not only does it help the "what's on the plate" illusion, but it also helps to increase the all too common lack of vegetable portions for the day.

A good idea is to chop up some of your favorite fresh vegetables, like spinach and tomatoes, and mix them into egg whites. You still get the flavor, texture, and emotional bond of "have to have" an egg. And you increase the volume of your egg meal with half the calories. Another good idea is to garnish the plate with some oranges or pineapples for added volume and a zesty twist. A hard-boiled egg is also a good choice. You can eat it whole or chop it up in a salad, creating the illusion of greater volume, as we saw with meats.

You can easily diminish the calorie issue with eggs by eating egg whites only. As Linda discovered, eating only egg whites can reduce the total number of calories with very little compromise of flavor. Still, you need to remember that, like everything you record on the FDL, whatever you eat has a number!

Short on fruits?

Not eating enough fruit is similar to not eating vegetables, but usually a lot easier to rectify. That is not the case, however, if you don't like *any* fruit or if the only fruits you do like are the high-sugar, high-glycemic-index fruits: watermelon, bananas, sweet grapes, mangoes, papayas, and pineapples. That doesn't mean these fruits are bad for you, but from a calorie count perspective, they will add up more quickly than apples, oranges, and pears.

If you research the fruit family, you will also see that many fruits have distinct nutritional benefits, which are good to keep in mind when addressing your specific health conditions. I strongly suggest you do this research as you try to rectify the lack of fruits in your daily diet.

Judy was always finding it tough to get to her target 120-calorie fruit number. She never was a fruit eater, and introducing fruits to her at forty-nine years old was proving to be difficult. More importantly, Judy had a chronic digestive problem and was always constipated. This health condition actually worked in her favor when suggesting what fruits she needed to add to her diet that would help her digestive issues. Still, she was not accustomed to just picking up an apple and eating it.

Fortunately, Judy bought into the idea of having a big, multi-food-source salad in the middle of the day. I suggested that she cut up some apples, papayas, and pineapples and toss them into her salad. This was the perfect solution to her fruit issue. In that one large salad she would get all the fruits she needed for her 120 target number. They also gave her natural digestive enzymes found in papaya and pineapple, which did wonders for her digestive system. And they added more variety to her salad, which increased her overall compliance.

If you're having difficulty getting to your fruit target number, doing what Judy did can be very helpful. Try to identify a few fruits that you like or can at least tolerate, and begin to mix them into your regular meals. For example, you can cut up peaches for your oatmeal, add pomegranates to your rice, dice up some pineapples and sprinkle them over your baked salmon, or simply cut up bananas and strawberries and add them to your cold cereal.

Some people ask me if making fresh fruit juices is a good alternative. Juicing is not a bad idea, but people who are not big fruit eaters usually have trouble sustaining the effort it takes to be a consistent juicer. This doesn't mean you shouldn't do it, but I would not recommend you spend $800 on a commercial-grade juicer. For those of you who have made fresh juices in the past, you know that the worst thing about juicing is the cleanup afterward. It takes five minutes to make a fresh glass of apple, carrot, and spinach juice, and it takes twenty minutes to clean your juicer afterward.

Another negative factor to juicing is that the pulp that is left in the juicer is much more nutritious than the juice itself. That means you are throwing away nutritious fiber, minerals, and vitamins that your body needs. Since you may already recycle your cans, bottles, and newspapers, you can understand when I say to recycle the pulp left in your juicer. Depending on what fruits and vegetables you used, you can learn to use the pulp to in preparing sauces for rice and pasta, as *chutney* (thick sauce of Indian origin) for meats and fish, or a flavorful addition to soups and gravies.

I believe that a better alternative to juicing is to make a smoothie with fruits and vegetables. You can purchase a high-speed blender at a reasonable price, and the smoothie lets you drink all the nutrients. In addition, the cleanup time is cut in half from that of a commercial juicer. The following chart shows how to prepare delicious smoothies that are nutrient rich and will help you meet your target goals for fruit and veggies.

DELICIOUS SMOOTHIES IN MINUTES

- Best fruits to use are apples, pears, pineapples, papayas, bananas, pomegranates, and assorted dark berries. These are high in vitamins, minerals, fiber, and other antioxidants.

- Best vegetables to use are the leafy green, nutrient-rich variety such as spinach, cabbage, and kale, or sprouts such as alfalfa and mung bean, which are a great source of A, B, and C vitamins. Of course, fresh carrots are always a favorite for flavor and color and are a good source of beta-carotene.

- Use a 2:1 ratio of fruit to vegetable, especially when you first try these drinks. The veggies may be a tad bitter, but the fruits will help mask them and make the smoothie easier to drink.

- Put enough water in the blender to just cover the fruits and vegetables, and blend on high for a few minutes or until you have the desired consistency.

- You can get adventurous by adding soy milk or almond milk instead of water. This will definitely make your smoothie a meal. Note: you may have to acquire a taste for this smoothie.

Another suggestion for using your blender is to make a flavorful thick vegetable soup. I make a broccoli rabe and asparagus soup that I think is delicious. Mix it with some onions, garlic, basil, and some peppers, and then warm it up on the stove.

Mastering your FDL

As you continue logging what you eat in your FDL, you will notice different trends in your caloric intake. These changes may be based on emotional influences, time constraints, social events, and unexpected personal obligations. When life happens, your objective is to navigate through these personal distractions, focusing on your target goals of balancing your food categories without going over your global target number.

One of the strengths of tracking and recording your foods often is that you will have a real-time account of where you are for the day. I have found this continual diligence to recording your food intake the best way to develop new and sustainable habits. There is an old saying, "Experience is your best teacher." I think it is more accurate to say, "Your *own* experience is your best teacher."

I believe the more intimately you are tied to the process, the more capable you are to take ownership, which results in the *process* becoming your new, healthy *habit*. I have observed that most diligent patients, committed to small incremental changes, reach a point where they have mastered the art of creating balance in their food intake by consistently logging their FDL. At that point they no longer need the FDL; time and repetition became their best teacher.

Creating an arc

Another task in mastering the FDL is to learn to create the "arc." An arc is a curve, or continuous part of a circle, used to specify the amount of food you should eat at certain times of the day. I have explained the need to eat more during more active times of your day and, conversely, not to eat during inactivity. The principle of the arc is to help you visually match your food consumption to the activity of your day. Earlier we discussed the need to spread your meals out during the day to avoid eating large meals that would spike your blood sugar levels.

At the bottom of the sample FDL, there is a list of percentages next to the Time column. These percentages represent the amount of caloric intake you should have during these times of day, assuming you are most active during the middle of the day. They represent the arc that defines your optimal quantity of caloric intake during the day.

You can modify this column to fit the activity levels of your day. The optimal goal is to eat your larger meals just before your busiest or most active times of the day, and your smaller meals when are less active. Physiologically, this helps your body consume the available blood glucose for energy instead of conversion to fat storage.

More tips for food substitutions

Food substitution is primarily done for the purpose of exchanging less desirable food choices for more healthy food choices; high-glycemic foods for low-glycemic (less sugary) foods; high-calorie, less nutritious foods for low-calorie highly nutritious foods. Not only will these exchanges improve your health, but they will also let you enjoy much higher energy levels.

For example, you are accustomed to eating a dinner that consists of a meat such as chicken, a starch such as potatoes, and a vegetable such as spinach. Your normal *preparation* has been fried chicken, fried potatoes, and creamed buttery spinach. Your original *portions* are three pieces of chicken, 2 cups of potatoes, and 1 cup of spinach. The object is to substitute foods, preparations, and portions from unhealthy to healthy without compromising the general food source or the amount of food consumed. This substitution will result in a lot less calories, a lot less toxins, and a lot more energy. Consider these healthy alternatives to your original meal:

- First substitution: Grill the chicken, bake the potato, and steam the spinach. To help you maintain incremental changes, only make one change at a time. Maybe just grill the chicken and leave the sides as usual.

- Second substitution: Make sure you take the skin off the chicken, which eliminates unnecessary fat calories, and switch to a sweet potato, which has a significantly lower glycemic index.

- Third substitution: Eat two pieces of chicken instead of three, 1 cup of potatoes instead of 2 cups, and increase the spinach to 2 cups instead of 1 cup. You can also include a

> green salad before the main meal to take up some stomach
> space and help with the "I'm full and satisfied" feeling at
> the end of the meal.

Following these suggestions and similar ones to make healthier choices of food and preparation, as well as reducing your quantities, will go a long ways to helping you succeed in your health goals. For more tips on how to make these powerful substitutions, see Appendix D.

Calorie exchange caution!

I do not mention this *calorie exchange* mechanism to my new patients; if not used correctly, it will violate the integrity of tracking your food intake in your FDL. Still, exchanging calories is recommended out of necessity for special circumstances; it is not to become a method of regular practice. Here's how the calorie exchange works.

Grains, breads, pastas, potatoes, fruits, and vegetables are all part of the carbohydrate family. The fundamental ingredients in all these foods are simple and complex versions of glucose. When the body breaks down the carbohydrate, it really can't distinguish the source from which it originated.

So, logically, your number of carbs can be *exchanged* between these food groups on your FDL. Scientifically, this logic is partially valid; practically, it can create a nutritional nightmare. For example, you dare not eat 500 calories of cake and say you're going to log the 50 calopoints like this: 26 in the carbs column, 12 in the vegetable column, and 12 in the fruit column. Mathematically, the 50 calopoints are recorded correctly for the calories you consumed, but nutritionally you are in *dietary disaster mode.*

Here are some suggestions for nutritionally sane calorie exchanging between the carb, veggie, and fruit columns. If you go over your target number in the fruit column, you can log the extra calories in the carb column, as long as you don't go over the carb target number. Similarly, if you go over your target in the carb column (eating potatoes, corn, or whole grains), you can log those extra calories in the fruit column. At least you have eaten nutritious foods, though in too great a quantity. Again, this exchange mechanism is not designed to be a daily alternative to let you indulge your "potato habit"; it is meant as a safety valve on the occasional mishap for daily calculations.

This calorie exchange can also work for the protein family, which includes meats, fish, beans, eggs, and dairy products. In your FDL, I separated the dairy from the rest of the proteins based on its lack of nutritional value and the potential for allergic reactions. If you occasionally go over your target for proteins, you can log your extra calories in the dairy column, and vice versa. Let me repeat, this exchange of calories should be occasional and not habitual. Most importantly, moving calories from one column to another is only viable if you don't go over the target sum of all the columns.

In the next how-to chapter we will continue discussing the positive power of moving your body. Simply put, you were born to move. Mastering this area of your wellness goals will enhance all your eating goals, improving the function of all the vital systems in your body.

Chapter 9

YOU WERE BORN TO MOVE!

C REATING A REGULAR unbreakable habit of daily exercise is by far the greatest personal discipline a person can achieve in their quest for physical fitness. It takes time, physical effort, and mental stamina to consistently work out regardless of how you feel, what the weather is, or even a change in the planetary alignment. I mentioned before that the methodology for creating a solid exercise routine is to start off slowly and steadily increase the time and intensity of the exercise over the weeks to follow.

With that goal in mind, your first exercise routine was the three minutes of abdominal crunches. Hopefully you have been doing this routine and are now prepared for the next incremental step in your exercise program. For some, it may be tempting to just cut to the chase and do the entire twenty-minute routine from the beginning of your wellness program. You might be saying, "What's the big deal? It's just twenty minutes." It may not be a big deal for some, but I believe that establishing new, lifelong habits are more important than just following a routine of exercises. Building a foundation of exercise for life is more prudent than just trying to get to the end of a short-term goal. So I'm assuming that, for at least the first week, you have done your three-minute crunches every day to the highest level of your present ability.

WEEK 2: PHASE 2 OF YOUR EXERCISE PROTOCOL

In Phase 2 of your exercise routine, your goal is to accomplish a four-minute set of lunges. (You can view these exercises on my website at www .schoolofwellness.com.) A *lunge* is a lower body exercise that targets the buttocks and leg muscles, including hamstrings and quadriceps. If done correctly, the following four minutes of exercise should be totally exhausting. Ready? Let's begin.

- Start in a standing position with your feet shoulder-width apart.

- Take a ¾-stride forward with your *right* leg.

- Hold both arms down at your sides with your fingers pointing to the floor.

- Then concentrate on bending your *left* knee straight down to the floor. As you bend your left knee, you will also have to bend your right knee. But the key to the exercise is moving the left knee straight down to the floor, in alignment with your left hand.

- Return to your starting position.

- Follow the same pattern with your right leg leading. Then alternate to complete the exercise.

Two points to note; it's OK for the left heel to come off the ground when bending your left knee. Also, it is critically important that you resist the urge to lean your body forward, which can cause a strain in the groin, hip flexors, and anterior hip. The degree to which you bend your knee toward the floor is based on the strength of your legs and the stability of your core muscles. Only go as far down as the strength of your legs will allow in order for you to get back up, and to the degree your knees can handle the pressure.

Also, if you feel unsteady, you may want to do the lunges holding on to a chair on each side at the beginning. Some patients do this exercise in a hallway where they can hold on to the wall. The key is to do this exercise slowly and steadily, concentrating on your balance and the proper bending of your legs.

Obviously, you don't need much room to perform this exercise as described. If you would like to get somewhat adventurous, you can lunge down a hallway in your house. Jacque has a little trouble with her knees, which has the tendency to throw off her balance when she bends into her lunges. So she does this exercise in a long hallway of her house. She starts at one end and basically lunges up and down the hall, moving forward to the other end of the hallway. This adds a little variety, plus she has the security of knowing she can always hold on to the wall for stability.

Once you have the technique down, use the following time structure to complete your four minutes of lunges:

- The goal is to complete four minutes of the lunge exercise, doing repetitive lunges for forty seconds, then taking a twenty-second break.

- Start exercising at a steady pace, paying close attention to form and balance. After forty seconds, stand up straight and take a deep abdominal breath, then exhale slowly.

- Rest in this standing position for twenty seconds, then begin the next set of lunges.

- Your goal is to do four sets of forty-second lunges with twenty seconds of rest between each. At the beginning, you should plan to complete the *time* goals, regardless of how many lunges you were able to do in each forty-second interval. Later we will set those goals as you improve your exercise capacity.

A note for beginners: Don't be fooled into thinking that the sixty seconds of rest during your four-minute routine will make it a breeze; if the lunge routine is done correctly, you'll be huffing and puffing after the second minute.

As you embrace the philosophy of slow incremental changes, you must be committed to completing both your three-minute abdominal and your four-minute lunge exercises *every* day during this second week of your program. That means seven minutes of your day must be set aside to accomplish these two exercise routines. When you have establish your seven-minute exercise habit, you will be ready to move on to the next phase.

WEEK 3: PHASE 3 OF YOUR EXERCISE PROTOCOL

Phase 3 of your exercise routine involves focusing on the upper body. The goal in the beginning is not to develop 20-inch biceps; it is to focus on toning, strengthening, and building endurance in the various upper body muscle groups. Earlier in the book we reviewed various methods of exercise that are designed to elicit different muscular outcomes.

During this first level of your exercise program, you must focus on correct movements and form. The last thing you want to do is to injure yourself because of improper form or from overdoing it. Don't try to make up for twenty years of being a couch potato in three weeks.

Exercise tips

There are five muscle groups you are going to target in Phase 3. Your goal is to exercise each muscle group for one minute; your total time will be five minutes for this beginning upper body routine.

This basic series of upper body exercises can be done with a light set of weights or an exercise band. If you are using weights, use wisdom in choosing them. Use poundage that is challenging but not so heavy that there is a risk of injury. You may have to adjust the poundage of the weights, depending on the exercise.

If you're using an exercise band, stand on the center of the band and hold on to each of the ends. Adjust the tension of the band by rolling it up in your hands for the appropriate tension for each exercise.

Also, it is a good idea to do these exercises in front of a mirror. As you watch your movements, you can make corrections and adjustments to your form.

Biceps

The first exercise focuses on the biceps:

- Stand with your legs shoulder-width apart.

- Slightly bend your knees and tuck in your abdomen.

- With your hands starting at your side, slowly bend your elbows and curl the weight or pull the exercise band upward toward your shoulder. Do this movement slowly and methodically. Don't jerk. There is no rush.

- Count three seconds up for the contraction and three seconds down to the starting position. This six seconds should allow you to complete ten biceps curls in one minute.

Triceps

The next exercise focuses on the triceps. This is the muscle group on the back of the upper arm that is responsible for allowing the extension of your elbow.

- Stand with knees slightly bent and abdominals tucked in.

- Bend your back slightly forward.

- Begin this exercise with elbows bent and both hands pressing on the back of your hips.

- Extend the elbows backward until your arms are straight back, slowly counting three seconds out. If you're doing this exercise correctly, your upper arm should be extended parallel to the ground (another good reason to do this exercise in front of the mirror so you can monitor your form).

- Then bend elbows slowly, bringing hands back to the hips, counting three seconds in.

Shoulders

The next exercise focuses on the shoulder muscle group. Be careful to choose your weight or the tension on the band correctly for this exercise. The stability of the shoulder weakens as you lift it to a parallel position to your body. It is advisable to use a lighter weight and less tension on the band in the beginning. This will avoid any risk of injury to your shoulder.

- Again, assume the usual starting position—knees slightly bent and abs tucked in.

- Begin with your hands down at your sides.

- Slowly lift your arms away from your body until they are perpendicular to it (forming a cross).

- Again, the same rule applies—three seconds up and three seconds down to your sides, slowly, with the end goal of ten repetitions in the sixty-second interval.

Back muscles

The next group is the back muscles. The starting point for this exercise is slightly different.

- Begin by tucking in your abdomen.

- Hold your hands directly in front of your thighs.

- Now bend your knees and bend your back forward at the same time so that your hands are now below your knees, about 8 inches from the floor. (If you're using an exercise band, adjust the tension by grabbing the band lower down so it's taut in the starting position.)

- Pull the weights or band directly up to your armpit and then lower them back down, using the same three-second count you used for the other exercises. You should complete ten repetitions in the sixty seconds allotted.

Chest muscles

The final group is the chest muscles. The starting position for exercising this muscle group is completely different from that of the other groups.

- Exercise band: Wrap the band around the highest part of your waist and tie it at the upper area of your abdomen, just below your chest. You may need to make the band tight to really feel the tension in this exercise.

- Lock your thumbs in the band and slowly pull the band away from your chest in the familiar count of three seconds out and three seconds in.

- Weights: With weights in hand, begin by lying on your back with your hands on your chest. Lift your hands toward the ceiling until your elbows are extended, then bring them back down to your chest, using the familiar three-second count. (If this is not challenging, you can substitute this exercise for the modified push-ups described later in the text.)

SUMMARY OF PHASE 1 THROUGH PHASE 3 EXERCISES

Let me clarify a few details regarding your exercise routine for the first three weeks before I discuss the advanced levels of the Genesis Diet exercise routine.

- These first three groups of exercises (total twelve minutes a day, seven days a week) should be committed to habit during the first three weeks of your program.

- There are no rest breaks between the three sets of exercises except for the twenty-second breaks built into the basic lunge routine. You will be exercising continuously for twelve minutes when you have mastered this new health habit.

- Never hold your breath while exercising. Concentrate on trying to inhale deeply from your abdomen. When you exert effort, you exhale. For example, time your breathing so that when you crunch your abs, raise from your lunge, or pull against the weights, you are exhaling.

ADVANCED GENESIS DIET EXERCISE ROUTINE

By the third or fourth week of exercise, you should be ready to increase the intensity of your exercise routine. As I have mentioned, your eventual goal is to get to twenty minutes a day of focused exercise and incrementally intensify each routine, creating an increased demand on each style of exercise.

Level 2

The next step is to get to Level 2 of your exercise routine. To do that, you simply increase the current twelve-minute routine to twenty minutes. (Tell me you love me.) For example, you will need to increase the abdominal crunches to five minutes, the lunges to five minutes, and then double up the upper body routine, for a total of ten minutes. You need to remain at this level for at least one week. Remember, you want to be safe, steady, and focused on building a permanent habit.

Level 3

Level 3 of your advanced exercise routine incorporates an assortment of variations of each exercise, which you can customize according to your own preference. The following is a review of each of these routines by phases that will allow you to test out the modifications when the time comes.

Modified abdominals

The basic level of abdominal exercise called for six seconds of contraction and brief relaxation between crunches. The advanced crunches have little to no breaks in abdominal contraction in its most intense routines. All the following exercises are done with the abs and pelvis in a locked position. This position is the posture you created when you initiated the crunch. Tilt the pelvis and bring the ribs toward the belt. 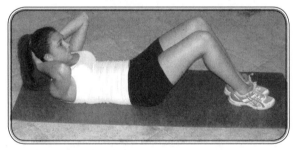 In the basic crunch exercise you relax after six seconds. In this advanced routine you remain in that locked position, abs contracted with pelvis tilted and ribs to belt.

Leg lift and stretch

Lying on your back with your hands at your side, slowly lift your legs above the floor about six inches. Make sure your legs are straight and held together. Next, with your legs still raised, bring your arms up and over your head and try to touch the floor behind you. Then slowly bring your hands back to your side. Do this as many times as you can for about two minutes. Remember to constantly hold the abdomen firm and the pelvis tilted so the lower back is flat on the ground. If you can't do this for two minutes straight, that's OK. Do it as many times or as long as you can, rest, and then continue. The point is, just don't give up. Eventually you will be

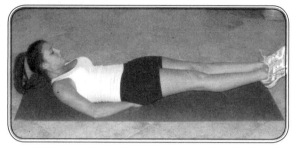

able to do this exercise and all the following exercises completely and smoothly.

Caution: If this exercise is too difficult to do, modify the position so it can accommodate your ability *without injuring your back*. This is not cheating; it is just a modification. Instead of keeping your legs straight out, bend your knees so your thighs are perpendicular to the floor, keeping feet off the ground. This will take some pressure off the abdomen and make it easier to complete the exercise.

Leg cross and hold

Begin this exercise in the same position as in the picture of the previous exercise, pelvis tilted up and ribs to belt with the abdomen contracted. Both legs are straight out and elevated about six inches off the floor. Then, bring one leg up to your chest and grasp your knee with both hands, continuing to pull it to your chest while the opposite leg is still extended six inches above the floor. Hold this position for about two

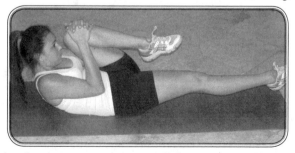

seconds and then release that leg, return it to its extended position, and hold; repeat movement with the opposite leg. The goal is to continue this exercise for a full two minutes. Like the previous exercise, do it as many times as you can comfortably, rest, and then continue.

To modify this exercise to your ability, keep your legs bent, never letting them extend all the way, while moving them six to twelve inches. The movement should be enough to feel the contraction of the abdominal muscles.

Torso crossover

Following the same basic pattern of the previous exercise, clasp both hands behind your head with elbows pointing out. Follow the same procedure of bringing one leg at a time toward your chest; then rotate the right side of your body so you can touch your right elbow to your left knee. Then reverse this pattern with the opposite elbow and knee. The effect is a crossover movement as you bring opposite elbow and knee together while constantly keeping the abdomen contracted. (For modification, please view video on the website at www.schoolofwellness.com.)

Full power stretch

Again, staying in the same basic position as the previous exercises, lift both legs off the floor about six inches and then bend both knees and draw them up toward your chest. Grasp knees with your hands, pulling them as close to your chest as possible. Then release your legs and extend them again to that position six inches off the floor, while stretching both your arms over your head until you touch the floor behind you.

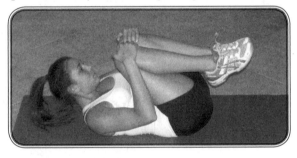

The modification version is similar to the previous exercise. Grab both legs and pull them toward your chest, then release them, but only allow them to go down to the point that you feel the contraction of the abdominal muscles.

Modified lunges

Modifying the lunges to increase the effectiveness of the workout may seem brutal in action but is very positive in a progressive training sense. I like to increase the intensity of the lunges in three stages. The only downside to the new levels of intensity is that some of the modified maneuvers may be difficult if you have a preexisting injury to the knees, hips, or lower back. I encourage you to access regular chiropractic care as you are completing the Genesis Diet program to assist in these situations.

The *first-stage* modification is to simply increase the length of time of the actual lunge exercise to fifty seconds, followed by a ten-second rest. Then add a twist of the upper body at the lowest point of the lunge. Take your three-fourths step forward and drop into the lunge position. When you reach your lowest point, hold it and twist your upper torso to the side of the forward leg. You can do this with your arms extended wide to maintain stability, using the wall or a chair for balance. You can also place your hands on your hips, which will force the engagement of more of the abdominal core muscles.

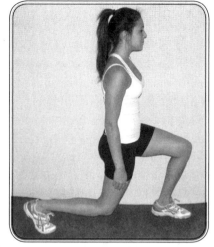

The *second-stage* modification involves increasing the holding time that you are at the lowest point of the lunge. When you reach the lowest point, either hold for six seconds (you may progressively build up to six seconds) or steadily bounce three or four times into the lunge. At the same time, contract the abs by twisting your torso as in the first-stage modification.

The *third-stage* modification uses a plyometrics technique to perform the lunges. You will need to be a little athletic to perform this maneuver, but if you can get this down... oh, what a workout! Just like the basic lunge exercise, you begin by stepping forward and dipping into the lunge position. When you reach the lowest point, you pause for a moment and then explode out of the lunge position, leaping into the air with both feet. You switch your leg position in midair and land in the opposite lunge position.

This technique may be a case of "you need to see this" rather than trying to figure out the written instructions. I admit, I did make it sound kind of dramatic, like it is some type of ninja move. In reality, it is a great exercise to eventually perform as you progress toward your fitness goals. When you are able to do five minutes of lunge plyometrics, you will know you are getting into fabulous shape. This one exercise combines endurance training, aerobic training, strength training, and power training. It will also improve your balance, coordination, and the stability of the joints in your ankles, knees, and hips.

Modification of upper body exercises

There are three ways you can step up the intensity of the upper body exercises. The actual maneuvers of the basic upper body routine remain the same, but the movements will change. You will need to refer to the basic exercises to compare these modifications of the upper body movements.

To increase strength

This will require longer counts for each maneuver. Bring the weight or exercise band to its maximum point of resistance in three seconds and then hold the tension at that point for another three seconds; finally, bring the weight back to a resting position (slowly) over a six-second count. For example, in exercising your biceps, bring the resistance to its maximum point by curling the weight or pulling up the band. (Be sure that your elbow is not in a locked, fully flexed position to avoid injury.) Count to three, and then slowly, over a six-second count, bring the weight or band down to a resting position. Repeat.

To increase endurance

In this situation, using light resistance, go through the upper body exercises in a rapid one second up and one second down one-two cadence. Theoretically, you can accomplish thirty repetitions per minute in each exercise. Even though this method is most notorious for creating an abundant amount of sweat, it will also increase muscle endurance and tone.

To increase power

This one is my favorite. In this exercise the exertion part of the exercise is done in a burst of energy, and the return or rest stage is done over the familiar three-second count. For example, to do the shoulder exercise, start with your arms in the usual "at your side" position. Then, suddenly burst your arms straight up to the side, count to three, and then slowly bring the arms down on a three count. This helps train certain types of muscle fibers to respond faster and stronger over a period of time. This is essential if you still have aspirations to participate in athletics competitively.

Remember, as you advance toward the optimal exercise routine, your ultimate goal is to establish a consistent and sustainable habit of daily exercise. As the routine becomes easier, you need to consciously increase the intensity to avoid complacency or boredom.

On the www.schoolofwellness.com website, you can preview the Genesis Life Seven Weeks to Wellness Program. This members' only page has several fifteen- to twenty-minute workouts to add variety to your exercise routines. It's acceptable to pick and choose the exercises you like and modify the routines to fit your personal goals. Just keep in mind that it is necessary to cover all the muscle groups. It is also important to alternate the type of exercises occasionally to assure a good mix of strength, endurance, and power training.

In the next chapter you will learn to address two foundational health factors that many wellness programs ignore. Without this understanding, you may find it difficult to achieve your optimal wellness goals. There is simply more to wellness than proper diet and exercise.

Chapter 10

ELIMINATING THE STRESS FACTOR

A T THIS POINT you have been given the tools you need to get into shape and the understanding of how to overcome obstacles and cultivate proper success attitudes to make that happen. Now I want to share with you two factors that will ultimately contribute to your success or impede it. I am devoting an entire chapter to this vital subject because I can honestly say it is the reason I wrote this book.

In earlier chapters I gave you an overview of the negative effects stress can have on your health. Now I want to share specifics with you of how to overcome the risks to your health goals that uncontrolled stress represents. The essence of my message to you for living in optimal health is embodied in your ability to overcome the health risks caused by the stresses of daily life.

As a chiropractic doctor, in my twenty-five years of helping patients succeed in their fitness goals, some foundational truths have become quite clear to me. One is that regardless of the how-to information you have, *if you cannot deal successfully with stress, you will not succeed in your fitness goals.* Another, which is closely related, is the vital importance of *maintaining proper balance to the spine,* promoted in part by developing good posture.

Diet and *exercise* have been the industry standard for marketing most health, weight-loss, and fitness products and programs. As we have discussed, these are critical factors to the achievement of your wellness goals. However, the foundational factors of overcoming stress and maintaining spinal health, while they are often popular health-related topics, are rarely given the same amount of attention as diet and exercise. As you discover ways to strengthen these two foundational factors to your optimal health, you will be more motivated than ever to pursue your long-term wellness goals.

There are a few things in life you just can't avoid. The old saying is, "You can't avoid death and taxes." Well, that's not necessarily true. With the right accountant, you can be a multimillionaire and still receive a tax refund. And if you are a Christian who believes in the soon return of Christ, you may be fortunate enough to avoid death and experience the "twinkling of an eye" transformation!

I think most people would agree that there is one thing that no one who lives on the planet can ever avoid: *stress*. In the following pages you will learn to recognize areas of stress that may be affecting your health. And you will gain understanding for eliminating stress and for keeping your nervous system functioning at optimal capacity. The fact is, *your ability to eliminate stress and maintain balance to the spine and nervous system are more vital to your overall well-being than any other aspect of wellness.*

> If you cannot deal successfully with stress, you will not succeed in your fitness goals.

THREE "FLAVORS" OF STRESS

There is no way to get around experiencing stress, especially since it comes in three "flavors": chemical stress, emotional stress, and physical stress. *Chemical stress* is primarily caused by the foods we eat and the beverages we drink. But it also includes the air that we breathe and our chemical intake through medications and the substances we put on our skin. These are only a few of the environmental stressors that affect your health.

The vital organs of the body such as the lungs, liver, kidneys, and even the skin are "stressed" when having to work harder to eliminate these toxic substances. Choosing to live a healthier lifestyle and being aware of sources of chemical stress to the body can help to mitigate its consequences.

Not as easily handled, perhaps, as the chemical stressors are the *emotional* and *physical* stresses that take their toll on our bodies, minds, and spirits. Because the Genesis Diet is an overall wellness program, based on biblical principles, it would be remiss not to address these life stressors that could hinder, and in some cases completely thwart, your ability to achieve your health goals. As I discussed briefly in earlier chapters, I believe emotional stress will motivate your actions more than any other factor in life. And physical stress will create neurological interference that, at a minimum, will cause physical pain; if not addressed, it can be the single most common cause of disease.

How hard can it be?

It would be so simple if all my patients were robots or if I practiced in the town of Stepford.[1]

I would give them instructions on the essentials of getting healthy, and, in their robotic way, they would just follow the directions perfectly. No complaints, no excuses, no distractions, just 100 percent compliance. But since that's not the case in the world of reality in which we live, I must address the truth of how people act and react to the stress around them.

I am sharing with you what I have learned in my chiropractic experience of helping thousands of patients over the last twenty-five years. While I'm not a psychologist, after many years of treating patients, I have identified emotional factors that prevent them from following my instructions and being successful.

For example, one of my patients, who showed great interest in getting into shape and improving her overall wellness, was showing little or no results from week to week. Soon after she started the program, she divulged that she was having trouble following some of the dietary instructions because of the lack of support from the people in her home, primarily her husband.

Over the next several visits, she was still showing little or no results in her weigh-ins, and her FDL was still chaotic. As she became more comfortable in sharing her woes with me, she told me that her husband was more than just not supportive. He was very critical and demeaning regarding her attempts to get into shape. The icing on the cake was the day she came in with a black eye.

Actually, she had been living with an abusive spouse for years. She felt trapped by his tyranny. Because she was uneducated, possessed no job skills, and felt she was too ugly to leave him and get a job to support herself, she stayed in that destructive relationship. She was beaten down and brainwashed by a sadistic bully. (He is lucky that she was not my sister!) In the end, God rectified the situation, and she was able to break free from that overwhelmingly stressful situation.

I shared this with you to illustrate that the power and influence of emotional and physical stress can at times be so overwhelming that, for people who are serious about establishing long-term wellness, it would be foolishness to avoid the topic. The better you understand the enemy, the more power you will have to defeat him.

In chapter 7 I gave you several assignments for your first week of your Genesis Diet program, including making an assessment of the relational stressors you can identify in your life. There I listed the most common relationships that can induce emotional and physical stress. The added discussion here should be helpful to you in completing that assignment.

UNDERSTANDING STRESS IN THE MARRIAGE

The relationship between a man and a woman, based in a special bond of attraction, was initiated by God when He created Adam and Eve. According to Scripture, this covenant relationship culminates in the sacred union of marriage:

> For this reason a man shall leave his father and mother and shall be joined to his wife, and the two shall become one flesh.
>
> —EPHESIANS 5:31

God designed mankind to enjoy this ultimate union, becoming one flesh as they fulfill the covenant of marriage. I have concluded that there are three basic elements required for the formation of a successful marriage:

1. The need to marry the right person

2. The husband's treatment of his wife

3. The wife's treatment of her husband

I would never lecture on a formula to find the right person to marry. But there is a simple rule for identifying the *wrong* person. Love is a crazy mystery, but covenants, such as marriage, are written in stone. According to the Scriptures, people of faith must marry people of faith. The apostle Paul declared:

> Do not be bound together with unbelievers; for what partnership have righteousness and lawlessness, or what fellowship has light with darkness?
>
> —2 CORINTHIANS 6:14–15

While the context of Paul's discussion is broader than just the marriage relationship, the principle of not being bound to an unbeliever in marriage applies. If you have a spouse who is "unequal" in his or her philosophy toward the Word of God, your marriage will have an unstable foundation that will affect all fundamental truths for the Christian.

For example, it would be impossible to refer to the Bible for advice if both spouses don't agree on the infallibility of the Word of God. Any relationship is in trouble when one party is a born-again believer and the other is not. That is especially true regarding the biblical role for husband and wife, taught clearly throughout the Scriptures. If you don't get the first element right, marrying the right person, there is great potential for destructive stress to take its toll on the relationship.

The second element for a successful marriage involves the husband's role, his treatment of his wife. According to the Book of Ephesians, the husband is to treat his wife as Jesus treated the church. He explains sacrificial love of Jesus, who "gave Himself up for her" (Eph. 5:25). Jesus was willing to lay down His life for the sake of the church; He proved it at Calvary. Paul clarifies further:

> So husbands ought also to love their own wives as their own bodies.
> He who loves his own wife loves himself.
>
> —EPHESIANS 5:28

There is no greater sacrifice a person can make than to lay down his own life for another. A husband who is walking in sacrificial love is willing to give up his own selfish desires for the well-being of his wife and family. This does not always guarantee an appreciative wife, but in the eyes of the Lord, the husband is serving God well by his obedience.

The third element needed in marriage is for the wife to assume her biblical role in the relationship. The apostle Paul gives instructions to her as well:

> Wives, be subject to your own husbands, as to the Lord.... As the church is subject to Christ, so also the wives ought to be to their husbands in everything.... Each individual among you also is to love his own wife even as himself, and the wife must see to it that she respect her husband.
>
> —EPHESIANS 5:22, 24, 33

I am aware of the controversy this passage of Scripture has caused in the church. But if you hear the whole counsel of Scripture, there should not be a problem. These verses, in context, are referencing a godly marriage of two believers. It does not teach that a woman should be submissive to any husband but a godly husband. There are many ungodly husbands who love to quote this scripture out of context. But a woman should only submit to the direction of her husband if he is hearing from God. A godly husband who is receiving the guidance of the Holy Spirit will always have the best interests of his family in mind. That trust and respect he has earned from his wife will be a solid foundation for a happy marriage.

For these reasons, the husband and the wife should be on equal grounds when it comes to their commitment to the gospel. When the Word of God remains the standard for all their actions and they try to resolve their problems according to the principles of Scriptures, their disagreements will be settled by God and not man.

COMBATING STRESS IN THE PARENT-CHILD RELATIONSHIP

Being a father of three wonderful girls, I feel I can speak confidently regarding the necessity of time involvement in a parent-child relationship.

There is no doubt that the nature of children can be frustrating to parents at times. And it gets more complicated with the increase in number of children and the complexity of their individual personalities. Regardless of these perplexities, it is vital for parents to invest time into the development of a healthy parent-child relationship.

All three of my girls have different personalities and interests. Without revealing their names, let me share that one of my daughters is easygoing, one is stubborn as a mule, and one is the personification of a "high-maintenance" child. In spite of their individual temperaments, my wife and I have determined to consciously work hard to invest the time needed to develop a powerful parent-child relationship with each one.

Just as important is their continuous Christ-centered education, communicated through word and example. The Bible is clear that we must raise our children in the principles and precepts of the Scriptures. Then, even if the child strays from the Lord, the Word teaches that the seeds we sow as parents (and grandparents) will eventually take root and bring the child back into the will of the Lord:

Train up a child in the way he should go, even when he is old he will not depart from it.

—PROVERBS 22:6

If you have children who are breaking your heart (stress with a capital S), don't give up on them. Pray for them, and continually minister to them in loving words and actions. God is faithful to His covenant promises, and He answers our prayers.

Another important factor is to continually be mindful that children are children. They will, by nature, try to stretch us to the breaking point over and over again. In those stressful moments, our reaction is key to the success and future behavior of how our children will treat their children. Here are some examples of healthy parental roles:

1. A parent is a leader and never an enabler.

2. A parent must show respect to earn respect.

3. A parent must discipline according to the infraction and not based on their own emotions.

4. A parent must keep promises (reward for obedience; discipline for disobedience).

5. *A parent must never provoke their child to wrath* (Eph. 6:4).

The key objective for both the parent-child and child-parent relationships is that the Word of God be obeyed by all. God will surely bless a covenant relationship, and the fruit of good seed is harmony in the house.

OVERCOMING STRESS IN THE CHILD-PARENT RELATIONSHIP

Let me address adult children. Your child-parent relationship does not end when you're sixteen, eighteen, or forty. As long as you have a parent or grandparent, you should actively work on deepening your relationship with them. Throughout your lifetime you will experience different phases of relationship with your parents. No matter what the phase, you should always esteem your parents and show them respect. The Bible promises a long life for those who honor their parents:

> Honor your father and mother...that it may be well with you, and that you may live long on the earth.
>
> —EPHESIANS 6:2–3

You may be thinking to yourself, "You don't understand; my parents were the most horrible people in the world." You may come from an abusive or neglectful situation, and all you care about is how far away you can get from it—and as soon as possible. That doesn't change the fact that they are your parents. If you can't develop a normal, healthy relationship, you can at least pray for your parents that they will come to know the Lord. It may be too late to have a "storybook" relationship with your parents, but it is never too late for them to experience His redemption.

While I cannot discuss the entire concept in depth here, I want to mention that the key to overcoming these hurtful situations, according to the Scriptures, is *forgiveness.* Choosing to forgive them will release the love of God into your heart to heal you from the hurt. You may not feel like forgiving; you may think they do not deserve forgiveness. No one does. But choosing to forgive sets you free from the destructive power of resentment, bitterness, and other negative emotions. That purposeful act of forgiveness will release you from the hurtful past.

HANDLING STRESS IN YOUR JOB SITUATION

My wife teaches fifth grade at a local New York City public school. Every day, when I pick her up from school I ask her the same question, "How was school today?" Would you imagine her response always being: "Wonderful!. All the children behaved, everyone did their homework, and no one had trouble with the new math program"? Not.

The truth is that no matter your occupation, there is going to be a level of stress inherently present. Complaining about work is probably the most talked about subject between adults. You might wonder, with all the complaining going on, why anybody would show up for work the next day. In short, your occupation is probably a source of stress, perhaps on some days more than others. Like every source of stress, there are several solutions available to you. We will discuss two possibilities:

1. Quit your job and get a new one. This option may generate the fear (stress), "How am I going to survive?" However, some job situations are so negative that this may be a valid consideration.

2. Follow the biblical injunction: "Whatever your hand finds to do, do it with all your might..." (Eccles. 9:10).

The first option is self-explanatory. The second will eventually show much return in the eyes of God. There is no doubt that some jobs just stink in every aspect. Yet you can enjoy the blessing of God when you obey His command to give thanks in everything (1 Thess. 5:18) and to do it as if you were doing it for the Lord (Eph. 6:7–8). Regardless of the potential stress, perform your job with joy, the same joy that you would if you were working for the Lord. It is the Lord who will honor your diligence, and He will open doors for a better career and eventually prosperity.

RESOLVING FINANCIAL STRESS

Of all the complaints I have ever heard, the one complaint I have never heard is, "I can't believe I have all this money; what am I going to do with it? I'm so stressed out." It is a *lack* of money that is a burden on almost everyone, no matter how much they earn.

An overriding theme that repeats itself throughout the Bible involves the principle of sowing and reaping. The apostle Paul states this principle precisely: "Do not be deceived, God is not mocked; for whatever a man sows, this he will also reap" (Gal. 6:7). In other words, whatever it is you need is the exact thing that you need to sow.

In the case of finances, as a Christian it is imperative for you to sow finances into the work of the gospel in order for God to release the blessing of finances back to you. The concept of tithing has been taught faithfully in many churches, though I understand that in recent times it has fallen into disrepute in some church organizations. Man's opinions do not change the covenant agreement of God for blessing those who obey His command to tithe and to give offerings:

> "Bring the whole tithe into the storehouse, so that there may be food in My house, and test Me now in this," says the LORD of hosts, "if I will not open for you the windows of heaven and pour out for you a blessing until it overflows."
>
> —MALACHI 3:10

The blessing of God's promises to those who obey His tithing covenant are almost too good to be true. Sometimes people who tithe think that the money they give is solely for the support of the church. That is only partly true. God's purpose for your giving a tithe is to give Him a reason to bless you, relating your obedience to the principle of sowing and reaping. When you sow finances into the fertile soil of the kingdom, you can expect to reap a harvest; God will bless the remaining 90 percent of your income more than you can imagine. And He will pour out blessings that you cannot contain.

The power of God's promise cannot be underestimated. There are only two times in the Bible where God challenges His people to test Him (prove Him) to see if He will fulfill His Word. So my challenge to you is to trust God and tithe! Placing yourself and your family under the blessing of God through obedience to His covenant of giving (which is broader than tithing) will be your key to resolving the stress of finances.

CONQUERING STRESS IN THE AREA OF HEALTH

This section embodies the *essence* of my book and my purpose for writing it. The stress caused by being sick is a persistent enemy that burdens every aspect of daily living. The purpose of this book is to give the reader hope that wellness is a blessing from God and that, as we choose to be obedient to the Word of God, we will achieve it. At the end of this chapter, following the Affirmation Section, I will expound on a passage of Scripture confirming the Lord's involvement with our desire for health. Read on and be blessed.

Physical stress and your spinal column

Probably the most influential of all the laws of physics on our lives and the one we most take for granted is the law of *gravity*. For some reason I loved my physics classes in college. I don't think it was my affection for calculus; I think it was more the practical experiments that showed the potential destructive forces related to these physical laws. (They might explain the multiple injuries I incurred as a youth in my attempt to be a bona fide daredevil!)

We all know that gravity is a relentless and unforgiving force when challenged. But did you know that gravity can also wreck havoc on the position, balance, and movement of your skeletal system, in particular the spinal column? The mainstream health care world rarely addresses this physical reality—except to admit that direct trauma can cause damage to the integrity of your spine and lead to back pain, neck pain, headaches, or radiating pain, as in the case of sciatica.

What these physicians tend to ignore is that there are dozens of other physical factors (beyond acute trauma) that can also affect the stability of the spinal column, disrupting the delicate spinal nerves that control the overall function of your body. The chart below shows a few examples of physical stresses that can cause detrimental effects to your spine and nervous system.

INJURY FROM PHYSICAL STRESSORS

- Poor posture: How do you sit when watching TV? How do you sit at your desk? How do you talk on the phone? Caused by being overweight.
- Hard physical demands at work: housework (the most traumatic I believe); lifting heavy objects, especially at the workplace
- Participation in sports
- Sleep positions, how you use pillows
- Past injuries: from falls; trying to get into shape; car accidents
- The trauma of being born and of learning to walk

As you can see from the chart, avoiding physical stressors throughout life that can potentially impair your spinal column is nearly impossible. That makes the chances of developing an imbalance in the positioning, movement, and stability of your spinal bones nearly 100 percent. The problem is aggravated by the fact that most people and a majority of allopathic (conventional) health care personnel dismiss spinal imbalances as nothing more than a "pain in the back." They often prescribe an "easy remedy" of an anti-inflammatory or common painkiller.

In fairness, severe and chronic conditions (meaning increased and unbearable ongoing pain) are given more attention in allopathic health care. From a conservative medical approach, a course of physical therapy may be recommended at first. However, if there is a derangement in spinal movement and position, traditional physical therapy will at best give temporary relief. Surgical intervention to address a damaged disk or a narrowing of vertebral spaces can create relief for a season, but rarely without future side effects. More importantly, their primary focus on spinal imbalance, pinched nerves, and slipped disk being solely associated with back pain is ludicrous and potentially deadly!

It is for this reason I am addressing the necessity of treating spinal health as a critical cornerstone to the achievement of overall wellness. Eating great and getting regular exercise and plenty of rest are all vitally important to getting into shape and preventing sickness. But if you ignore an obstruction to the transfer of information from the brain to your muscles, organs, and glands (neurological interference), all the good food, rest, and gym time will do very little to prevent disease.

Consequences of neurological interference

In order to understand the possibilities of neurological interference, it will help to review in some detail the anatomy of the supporting structures of the nervous system. For example, the brain is encased and protected by a solid hard bony structure called the skull. The spinal cord, which is connected to and actually is an extension of the base of the brain, extends out from the skull through a passage way called the "foramen magnum." The spinal cord then proceeds through another protective encasement of bones called the spinal column, which is made up of twenty-five individual bones located from the base of the skull to the base of your spine.

Unlike the skull, the spinal column is very flexible and allows for a multitude of movements and positions that are necessary for daily life. Unfortunately, built into the wonders of spinal movement is the inherent opportunity of accidental injury or overuse that can compromise its function. In the same way that movement is of great benefit to your body, it can also harm it. Over-movement, directionally abnormal movement, or abusive movement can cause a positional or functional aberration to the spinal column.

For example, excessive external forces or persistent low-impact stresses to the spinal column can cause individual spinal bones (vertebra) to move out of their normal anatomical position and functional movement. As a result, this abnormal moving "bone-out-of-place" can very easily put pressure on and cause irritation to the delicate spinal nerves that exit from the spinal cord between these individual vertebrae.

Nerve interference from a misaligned vertebra is called a *vertebral subluxation*. You may be asking one or two questions at this point: "Is this a promotion for chiropractic care?" And, "Are you saying that pinched nerves can cause other health problems besides back pain?" The answer to both these questions is YES! Before I fully address your questions, let me continue with an explanation on how vertebral subluxation occurs.

The wisdom of God's design

If you believe the Bible, you know that God is the creator and designer of your physical body. My theme verse for my Genesis Diet program is Genesis 1:26: "Let Us make man in Our image, according to Our likeness."

When God designed man, He had a specific plan for each function of the body. When your body was developing in the embryonic stage, the first structure formed was the brain and nervous system. This is not a chance happening. We now understand that the reason God causes the brain and its nervous system to develop first is for this structure to function as the master control system for the rest of your development as a fetus; it is the actual seat of life.

As the nervous system develops, vital organs are connected to nerve endings, and the body continues to grow. Eventually, the nervous system is encased in bone (the skull and vertebra), which is designed for its protection. What godly wisdom in His design to protect these important, delicate structures! As a result of God's incredible wisdom, we observe a marvelously constructed human being in which the brain and nervous system act as the master control system for life. That also means that any interference to the flow of communication from the brain through the nervous system to any of the organs, muscles, or glands in the body will result in a malfunction of those body parts.

In God's wisdom, He also placed an early warning system within our bodies to indicate a potential malfunction. When there is nerve interference anywhere in the body, it registers *pain*. Unfortunately, when the remedy for pain is to mask it with pharmaceuticals, the nerve interference persists and may even worsen. This physical reality creates the basis for the chiropractic profession's claim that you should not wait for pain to see your chiropractor. Regular checkups will go a long way in support of the overall well-being of your health.

Paying attention to your body's signals

When you understand the vital role of your nervous system, you can see why a pinched nerve can cause much more than just back pain. If there is interference or pressure on a nerve, it will cause every signal in that nerve to be altered from the normal flow of neurological signals. Some of the signals are sensory receptors whose job is to indicate pain. Others are for motor function of skeletal muscles responsible for physical movements. Nerve interference in these areas will cause weakness and atrophy (deterioration) of the muscle to which it corresponds. Many fibers in the spinal nerves are concerned with the operation of the organs and glands of the body. If they experience interference and abnormal signals, the result will be abnormal function of the affected organ or gland.

This issue of nerve interference is potentially a severe threat to the overall health of a person. To take this concept a little further, I would recommend that everyone undergo a spinal evaluation (similar to that of a dental checkup) as a routine health measure for wellness and early detection of spinal imbalances. A body free of nerve interference will always function better than a body with nerve interference.

The spinal solution

When we focus on the function of the spinal column as it relates to your nervous system, it seems almost impossible to avoid trauma to this vital physical structure. There are so many situations, as I showed in the previous chart, that can cause the vertebrae to misalign and lead to nerve interference and/or a spinal subluxation.

I personally believe there is only one solution to correcting this problem of misalignment: everyone needs to have his or her spine checked by a reputable doctor of chiropractic. I realize some people still proclaim that they don't believe in chiropractors. Let me counter by saying there is nothing to believe in. It is not a profession that is based "on faith." It is a profession that requires the same amount of general medical education as required for other doctors before receiving training specializing in the care of the spine.

Let me end this discussion by presenting a two-sentence "infomercial" for chiropractic care. Traditional chiropractic care has proven its effectiveness in the less invasive treatment of back pain and other spine-related ailments, such as sciatica and tension headaches. It also addresses many more possibilities for promoting wellness than meets the eye. The following diagram shows the reality of the *cause* factors for most illnesses:

Physical stress→ Spinal subluxations→ Nerve interference→
Malfunctioning body parts→ Sickness and disease

If you need help finding a doctor of chiropractic in your area, visit my website at www.schoolofwellness.com.

Chapter 11

THE EXPERIENCE OF OTHERS

I N YOUR JOURNEY to get into great shape, you have learned that, before beginning, you must become *spiritually* and *mentally* prepared in order to create a strong foundation for long-term success in achieving your wellness goals. You understand also that there is no "magical jump-start program" on this journey, but rather a slow development of steady incremental changes over a long period of time. Finally, you have previewed the science, procedure, and formula presented here to create optimal natural wellness.

Theoretically you have arrived. You have the formula for your wellness program, and you know the pitfalls to avoid and the process for getting the accountability support you need for success. In these last two chapters I will give you two other helpful, perhaps even necessary, tools to insure your success. First, you can learn much and be strengthened to complete your goals by listening to *the experience of others.*

I would love say that I have had 100 percent compliance from all of my patients. In reality, it would be delusional for me to believe that the Genesis Diet program is so persuasive that every single person is able to succeed. In spite of that, I still believe that every person who wants to get well can get well. My challenge is to create enough positive leverage to move patients past the point of their excuses, past the point of their hindrances, and past the point of their complacency.

As I discussed in chapters 1 through 3, knowing *what* to do and *how* to do it is helpful. But unless you have the spiritual, mental, and intellectual foundation for *why* you are doing it, your success is in doubt. It is like the parable Jesus taught about the house built on sand that fell when the wind and rain came. He warned that we must build our house (our lives) on the rock, a solid foundation, to preserve them (Matt. 7:26–27).

The following stories of real-life struggles and successes of patients will serve you as great instruction and greater inspiration to triumph in your own quest for health. I believe that, beyond theory, your best learning tool is testimony of personal experience; it is wisdom that can help you to profit from the experience of others.

JUSTIFYING BAD HABITS

On occasion I have treated patients with a certain personality trait that is hard to describe though easy to recognize. They are fun-loving, sincere people who give the impression they are really enthused about getting into shape and making their positive lifestyle changes—except that they never make any changes; they just make smiley-faced, apologetic "I will try harder next week" excuses. These are always followed by the justification of why they couldn't do what they had to do because of some "convincing fairy tale" they believed to be a legitimate reason. Are you following me?

Nellie is a fun-loving, highly motivated, energetic always-on-the-run woman who acts and looks half her age. At first you would think that she is the perfect patient; I thought so too—except for that one attribute that seems to be counterproductive to the program: being "always on the run." Nellie's busyness was her foundational justification for every excuse she made regarding her failure to comply.

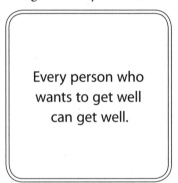

Every person who wants to get well can get well.

I would look at her half-filled-out FDL and scratch my head. There would be weeks where she would eat out at restaurants four or five days in a row because she was traveling to six different cities attending fund-raisers, visiting friends, or going to the rescue of some lost soul. When it came to doing her exercise, of course she had the "I was traveling" card. And when she was home, she pulled the "I'm doing construction in my house" card.

Every week there was someone's birthday she was organizing or some event that needed her utmost attention. After a while I found it odd that she never missed her appointments, never indicated she wanted to quit, and always justified her actions. In addition, she swore she would try to do better next week.

One day Nellie brought in her friend Ralph, who recently was injured. Ralph also needed to get into shape, and ideally, this friendship could be a great situation except that Nellie was the worst role model. However, one attribute of Nellie, previously undiscovered, suddenly came to my attention: Nellie was a *natural nurturer*. That's why she was running all over the planet; she honestly felt she needed to take care of everyone.

Now here was Ralph, right there in front of her and in front of me. Capitalizing on this newly discovered need to nurture, I added fuel to that fire. I charged her that it was her responsibility to make sure that Ralph got into shape, a responsibility that she gladly said yes to. The fact that Ralph urgently needed to work on his health situation was also a help. In the end, Nellie's commission to rescue Ralph was the single greatest influence for getting herself on track with the program. Her justification for failure stopped when she was needed for someone else's motivation to success.

Maggie was another "self-justification expert." She happened to become friendly with Nellie. Maggie's situation was a little different from Nellie's. She was a department head at the company where she worked. She had tons of responsibility and was truly busier that the average person. The problem was she was so busy that she never realized how busy she was. Everything she ate was either made for her or she bought it on the run. She reasoned that her job, which required that she walk miles a day in the hospital, was surely enough exercise.

Maggie's justification was more of an admission than an excuse. Her response to not meeting her weekly program goals always started with, "I know...but this is what happened," and would end with, "I know better and I will work on it for next week." Maggie definitely needed to get into shape. She had no present health emergencies, but she did have every marker of an impending disaster, including a significant family history that made her a candidate for a sudden health crisis.

Maggie would speak frequently about her weekend routine of relaxation she had with her husband. Even though she was close to retiring, she would never talk about it. One day I asked her, "What are you going to do when you retire?" Her response was quite appropriate: "Well I guess my husband and I will do what we do on the weekends every day." This was my opportunity to "drop the hammer" on her typical behavior. I said, "Maggie, if you don't start seriously taking care of the small things I'm teaching you now, you will never be able to enjoy the big things later." My warning seemed to get her attention. I continued, "In order to enjoy life, you must first choose life!" What Maggie needed was a better idea of what she could *have* and what she could *lose*.

Sometimes in the busyness of your business you forget to look at the big picture. Work is important, but it can become a justification for long-term failure on a larger scale. If you find yourself justifying your negative actions or even your lack of positive actions, you need to stop immediately and take inventory. Can your actions be beneficial or destructive for those around you? Will your actions in the present assure a good level of health and happiness ten or fifteen years from now? Those important considerations will inspire you to cultivate a healthy lifestyle in the present that you can carry into the future.

Moses made many powerful statements that are recorded in the Scriptures. But the one that rings in my head as one of his most powerful declarations is, "I call heaven and earth to witness against you today, that I have set before you life and death, the blessing and the curse. So choose life in order that you may live, you and your descendants" (Deut. 30:19).

GETTING ENOUGH VEGETABLES

As I discussed earlier, eating enough vegetables is probably one the hardest obstacles to overcome in the entire program. Though it is not an emotional or spiritual issue, it is a habit instilled deeply in our environment and culture. Even if you are originally from a foreign country where fresh fruits and vegetables are culturally eaten as part of the daily menu, after living a few years in America you will probably replace healthy "green and steamed" with "yellow and fried."

Mrs. C was originally from one of the island nations. At her first consultation she told me how she loved all kinds of vegetables. When she was younger, her grandfather had a vegetable farm, and she would help him during the harvest. She seemed very encouraged and confident that the dietary changes she needed to make were not too far from what she was used to eating. The dichotomy in what she said was a blaring dichotomy to what I was seeing. Mrs. C was more than 150 pounds overweight. My compassionate mind wanted to believe her insistence in her love for vegetables, but my educated mind said, "She hasn't eaten a salad in years."

As it turned out, her first FDL was severely lacking in the vegetable column. She couldn't understand why, saying that she was too busy that week to shop or prepare her meals. After a few weeks of consistent lack in the vegetable column, however, it didn't take her long to admit that, even though she loved vegetables, she seemed to unconsciously eliminate them from her diet. If you feel that this is your area of demise, let me reassure you that the solution is not far away or painful to achieve.

I made two suggestions to Mrs. C that almost immediately corrected the problem. The first was to create a bucket every day, as we discussed earlier, and to make sure that by the end of the day the bucket was empty. The preparation part became a bit of challenge for Mrs. C in the beginning. It was nothing that couldn't be solved by an *intentional* grocery shopping trip once a week.

The second suggestion was to do a one- or two-day vegetable fast every five days. This concept may sound weird, since a fast normally means to eat nothing at all. However, I am using the term, which is becoming popular in many circles, to indicate fasting from everything *except* a certain category of food; i.e., in a vegetable fast you eat only vegetables. It was not too long after this conversation that Mrs. C was on track for successfully reaching her health goals. Her weekly vegetable-only-fasts were a great way to reintroduce her to eating the greens she had loved. It was also a wonderful boost in moving the scale in a positive direction for her weight-loss goals. Before long the bucket was a daily habit, and she still continues the habit of eating only vegetables one day a week.

Mrs. C's original affection for vegetables was a help to reestablish her habit for eating them, but that is not always the case. Karen was a middle-aged woman who appeared to be in good shape. She wasn't overweight, and her body fat was in the acceptable range. However, she was very concerned with her family history of heart disease and diabetes. She had attended one of my lectures at her sons' school. What motivated her to come to my office was my explanation to the audience that poor diet and spinal subluxation can lead to sickness, even if you look like you're in good shape. I added, "This is especially true if you have a family history of certain diseases."

Karen was an especially difficult patient because she was convinced she didn't like any fruits or vegetables. In a situation like this, I am left with only two options and one motivating factor. Regarding motivation, I know that changes have to be made in the way she eats because disease that is self-induced by poor dietary choices is not an option for her; family history will become an issue. This reasoning, though valid, does not easily create the leverage she needs to pursue wellness goals because she looks good, feels good, and has no medical markers to indicate that she's in any imminent danger.

I needed to capitalize on some aspect of Karen's personality that would assist her in her journey toward compliance. I noticed that Karen perceived herself as being very influential to the people around her. Many people looked up to her because she was active in leadership positions in several social settings. She was the PTA president in two of her children's schools, she ran a woman's group at her church, and she was always helping out with various community functions.

Karen was a remarkably humble person who had the ability to influence many people. Observing this positive attribute, I told her that because many people looked up to her, she would be doing them an injustice if she were unable to continue in her public service as a result of sudden illness. In addition, I suggested that if she made positive lifestyle changes, she could be a great inspiration and motivator to the people she touched on a daily basis. This passion to serve others along with the disturbing thought of being unable to serve others was enough of a motivating factor to change Karen's thoughts about eating fruits and vegetables.

Now that there was a solid motivation in place, I was able to offer Karen two options. The first was, instead of trying to find fruits and vegetables she liked, to focus on those she was able to tolerate. We found out that plain salad, tomatoes, and cucumbers were tolerable. So every other day she made a 4-cup bucket of those three vegetables. Boring indeed, but the motivation behind the action was greater than the action itself, so she did it. That helped resolve the vegetable dilemma.

The second option was to become the "master of disguise." Karen loved her rice and beans. It took some convincing, but eventually I got her to convert to rice and peas. She also liked soup. So she started loading her soups with peas, carrots, and finely chopped broccoli. Fruits needed the "master of disguise" technique in a big way. Spreading peanut butter (not the best choice) on her apples and mixing pineapples in her yogurt were a beginning point for eating fruits. Over time, these and other changes became part of new habits that seamlessly evolved into her new lifestyle. For Karen, the principle of slow incremental changes over a long period of time prevailed.

Making Effective Substitutions

I discussed earlier some simple ways to substitute the unhealthy foods you like with a healthy version. (See also Appendix D.) For example, eat whole-wheat breads and pastas and brown rice instead of their white versions. Perhaps these real-life stories will illustrate how effective substitutions to promote your health goals can be easily made.

Estella was very motivated to achieve her optimal wellness goals because of a serious health issue. For a number of years she was borderline for developing a life-threatening disease. As a result, she actively researched healthy food choices and made them part of her daily life. Whatever could be substituted she would substitute. She is an example of how proper motivation can help you "give up" your taste/texture preferences for unhealthy foods and develop new tastes for foods that will keep you well.

The key to substituting foods effectively is to acquire a liking to the taste and texture of the new food; that will require the pseudoscience of slow incremental steps toward substitution. (My invention?) Practicing this science of slowly becoming accustomed to small, healthy changes in your eating habits has worked for my patients for years, without benefit of clinical data to prove its effectiveness. Who needs it? Success vindicates this approach to long-term wellness.

Juggling the Food Columns

In chapter 8 I discussed the legitimate mechanism for exchanging some amounts of calories between certain columns. I cautioned you to use this mechanism carefully so that you do not violate the workable principles for your FDL.

Terri was the master juggler. At times I thought she spent more time figuring out how to trade her calopoints between the columns than she did managing other aspects of the program. For example, she wasn't much of a protein eater but she loved her cheese. There were days that her entire protein allotment was calculated from the calorie overage in the dairy column. If done continually, her excessive dairy consumption (and lack of protein consumption) could become a body chemistry problem for her metabolism. Fortunately, Terri gained a balance and became the master juggler who was able to manage an excellent exchange of foods from category to category.

She has been able to help other patients with her creative exchange ideas that serve as effective compromises without violating the overall protocol.

Terri learned to make many of her exchanges between the dairy and protein columns and between the fruit and carbohydrate columns. She learned not to do it in excess, and she tapped into the tremendous flexibility available for managing your overall diet while still reaching your optimal wellness goals. If you learn to exchange calopoints carefully on an occasional basis, you will have nothing to worry about. It will serve you as a customizing of your particular preferences and help you toward your goals.

THANKSGIVING DINNER

This section could have been titled Christmas dinner, Easter dinner, Mikey's wedding, or the Fourth of July bash. You get the drill. Everyone needs help to reconsider the habitual feasting you have probably been doing since childhood. Big Ray, whom you met earlier in the book, is my best example of how to manage the gigantic family food feast.

A week or so after Big Ray gave me the news that he had lost twelve pounds, the calendar indicated that it was three days before Thanksgiving. Unfortunately, Ray was motivated to living up to the "big" in Big Ray. He reasoned that he deserved to indulge on Thanksgiving because he had been good for so many weeks. The "old Ray" was trying to barge in on the "new Ray." I was concerned and decided to give my counsel, hoping his commitment to accountability would kick in.

Surprisingly, it did not take much to convince Ray that we (both of us) would hate to see him create a regrettable situation and undo all the new habits that had taken us so long to establish. Ray rapidly and uncharacteristically (for the old Ray, that is) consented to a plan that would help him navigate these dangerous waters. It would allow him to taste all the delicacies of the dinner without violating any parameters he had molded into his new habits.

I broke the "feast" down into three sections: The *appetizers*, the *main course*, and finally, the potentially disastrous *dessert*. We made a covenantal agreement on adopting the plan and shook hands on it in the presence of Delores, his wife. The great thing about Delores was that she was 100 percent on my side. If Ray strayed from the plan by one extra fork of stuffing, she would rat him out in a heartbeat. Here is the plan.

The appetizer

The *appetizer* is divided into two helpings (plates) of food. The first plate must be only veggies: raw carrots, broccoli, celery sticks, etc. The second plate can be whatever you like as long as it is *half the size* of the vegetable plate. This will require that you manage your intake volume. The more delicacies you want to eat, the more you will need to precede them with twice that amount of vegetables. The rationale is simple; it is impossible to overindulge on the savory cheese puffs without loading up on the more filling (and healthy) vegetables first.

The main course

For the *main course* of your feast, you follow this same methodology. Before filling your plate with feast food, you need to eat 2 cups of green salad, then wait five minutes before you dig in to the main course. This plan requires some time management.

Ten minutes before the actual dinner is served, begin to eat your salad. That will give you time to spare before digging in to the main course. This helps in at least two ways: the salad fills more stomach space, and the time between courses allows the blood glucose levels to slowly rise from eating the appetizers and salad. The goal is, of course, to create a sense of fullness during the meal—especially by dessert time.

After eating your salad, you can eat as much of the main course as you want *as long as half the plate is always green.* As long as you fill half your plate with vegetables, you can eat as much turkey, stuffing, etc., as you can fit on the other half of the plate—again, managing your volume intake while enjoying all the holiday tastes.

The dessert

The dessert is perhaps the most "sinister" threat to blowing your food intake goals. Again, the plan is to manage the volume: Eat twice as much fruit as cake. Let the natural sweets satisfy your taste while indulging moderately in the potentially disastrous sugary sweets.

You may be saying, "Wow, that was a lot of food you had Big Ray eating." Well, he was not called Big Ray for nothing! I knew the dessert would be the most difficult test for Ray. In the end he was successful. He told me that he cut up an apple and put it in one plate, then took a forkful of various desserts to exactly half the volume of the apple slices. Brilliant!

THE POWER OF ACCOUNTABILITY

I hope I have convinced you that stress is the deadliest enemy you face, and probably the single most significant factor for causing failure in any self-help program. Stressful events such as a sudden crisis, deaths in the family, loss of a job, sickness of a loved one, or financial reversals threaten to sidetrack you from your health goals. Even joyful events like weddings or prolonged holidays can be factors that cause you to fail.

Let me repeat once more that the key to your long-term success is to slowly, incrementally break old habits and replace them with life-giving habits that result in optimal wellness. And remember that stress is an unavoidable foe. The only remedy to overcoming it is to build a strong foundation of repetition of good habits along with a steadfast commitment to be accountable.

Alma is my model patient in this area—not because she has more or less stress than the next person, nor is she a magnet for misfortune. She has excelled in becoming accountable; she is totally accountable to my coaching and (hopefully) to my desire to guide her to lasting success. Alma has lost most of the weight she wanted to lose, she regularly exercises, her spine still hurts, but not nearly as bad as it did before we met. And her blood chemistry issues are back to normal.

With all this success, she still never misses her appointments. Alma has plenty of responsibilities and opportunities to be sidetracked by stressful situations. Yet she has not allowed them to make her slip back into her old habits. Her rationale is simple and quite flattering to me. She believes that our visits are anchors that bring her back to the focus she needs: why she worked so hard to get into shape in the first place. At her appointment with me, it is not uncommon for to say, "Doc, this was a rough week. I'm not sure how well I did, but I knew I had to come to get myself back on track." That is the safety in accountability.

Finding a Genesis Diet doctor or other strong accountability partner is critical to your success, especially to conquer potentially devastating effects of stress. Becoming accountable also involves taking responsibility for your own actions. Never blame another person for your actions or justify the persuasion of another to cause you to slip. Being accountable will always keep you grounded to a source of positive influence. My hope is that long after you finish this book, you will refer to it as a helpful manual for your wellness program. You can also continue to frequent the www .schoolofwellness.com site as a source of positive inspiration and help for your health goals. The Weekly Focus section found there contains ideas to continually empower you to overcome the distractions of daily stress.

PREPARATION + OPPORTUNITY = SUCCESS

Bobby Unser, winner of the Indianapolis 500 three times, declares as his motto: "Success is where preparation and opportunity meet."[1] Opportunity alone does not guarantee success without its powerful component: *preparation*. The fact is that *intentional preparation* is vital for your success in any area of life. If you leave your day to chance—what you will eat, when you exercise, how you feel, required activities for the day—you are destined to encounter serious distractions from your health goals. It is undeniably true that my most successful patients are the ones who intentionally prepare for each day. The more areas of your day you can intentionally prepare for and plan, the more marked will be your rate of success. Many of my patients have caught on to this principle. Dianna came to mind immediately to use as an example to inspire you to prepare for your day.

Dianna needed to lose a modest amount of weight. More importantly, she was diagnosed with several metabolic syndromes for which she had to take medicines. Dianna hated taking the drugs. Understanding their side effects and just the thought of knowing that they were simply covering up the symptoms left her feeling frustrated. She was left with a sense of hopelessness for getting healthy again and back to her active lifestyle. She felt that her condition was robbing her of the joy of living life to the fullest. Needless to say, Dianna was very motivated when I told her there was hope to do just that.

At first she struggled, like most patients new to the program, with designing a schedule that would work with her daily routine. I told Dianna what I tell hundreds of patients: "Don't let the day run you; you need to run the day." Many people who

> Opportunity alone does not guarantee success without its powerful component: preparation.

do my program have tried other more commercial programs and failed, including Dianna.

Avoiding the hazard of quick fixes

Some of these commercial programs take the *preparation* factor out of the equation by making available a huge selection of preprepared foods. At first this sounds like a brilliant idea. You don't have to shop (except to buy the frozen dinner), prepare, cook, or even clean up your kitchen after the meal. Just buy a dozen frozen meals, pop them into the microwave, eat them, and throw the empty carton in the garbage. What can be easier than that?

According to these weight-loss protocols, it doesn't really matter how nutritious the meal is, or if the combination or portions are ideal, or even if it tastes good. What matters is simply that the calorie count is low; after all, losing weight is the ultimate goal. People who follow these lose-weight-quick programs must realize they can't do this forever. Their rationalization seems to be, "I'll just do this until I get back to my ideal weight. Then I will simply continue to eat healthily."

The sad fact is that this is rarely the outcome. How could it be? If, for some reason, you have the self-discipline (uncoached) to eat 180 prepackaged microwavable meals (which is highly unlikely) over a two-month period of time, what does it mean that you happen to lose eighteen pounds? Honestly what have you learned about eating healthy meals? What have you learned about shopping, preparing, and organizing meals that will meet the nutritional demands needed for optimal health? The answer is, *nothing*!

For this reason many people fail in their weight-loss goals, gaining the weight back that they lost, plus additional pounds. There was no foundation established for maintaining health, no accountability, no taking of ownership or establishing healthy habits. Nothing of lasting help for their health was learned.

I can't even begin to tell you how many patients, including Dianna, have told me the same or similar stories of their quick-fix fantasies. Dianna was not going to let that happen again. She bought into the *intentional preparation* idea hook, line, and sinker. Every day she set out the three water bottles she planned to drink that day. She left her supplements next to her nightstand to make sure she took them. Every third day she cooked enough whole grains and steamed vegetables to last for three days. She perfected the bucket concept, using many creative ideas.

Dianna also had her exercise times set daily, which could not be broken. And she never missed her appointment at my office. (She actually referred many more patients to my practice.) Her somewhat natural affinity to preparation easily became part of her new lifestyle habits. Her intentional preparation and hard work all paid off. She lost the weight she wanted to lose and was able to eliminate the need for the two medications that were causing her to despair, both physically and emotionally.

THE DP TEMPLATE

I have been continually amazed over the years at the creative ways my patients modify their use of the FDL. Even though I believe I have been thorough in the explanation of the FDL, some patients always add ideas to make the use of it more fun, interactive, and flexible.

Do you remember Denise from chapter 3? She was the patient who took the sample completed FDL to heart in the most serious way. For the first two weeks of her program, she ate only the foods listed in that sample FDL every day. I tried to explain to her that the sample was just that, a sample for use as a training tool to manage the calopoints numbers; I never intended anyone to use it as a continuous menu for the week.

She countered that the sample menu helped her to calculate the number of calopoints she needed in each column for each meal. The result: a simple new formula was born, which we call the DP template. This simple formula, based on the numbers in the columns of the sample FDL, helps you calculate appropriate quantities of substitutions you can use for those specific categories. For each meal, there is a number of calopoints in the appropriate columns that does not change.

For example, in the sample menu, the third meal has 14 points in the protein column, 6 in the vegetable column, 5 in the fruit column, and 4 in the butter and oil column. The basis for the DP template is to simply leave those numbers in the columns indicated (the sample is based on a 1,200-calorie menu), then place the substitution foods in their correct portions into the section corresponding to their description section.

THE DP TEMPLATE

- Meal 1: 12 points in the carbohydrate column. Eat any combination of carbs that stays within that 12-point limit. In this case the variety may be limited, but you still have a numerical basis for diversity. A different hot cereal, a cup of dry cereal, or slice of toast may fit the parameters.

- Meal 2: 5 points in the fruit column and 12 in the dairy. Again, you can easily substitute for different fruits, substitute an egg for the dairy, and exchange the points for protein for later in the day. You can even swap the first and second meals a few times a week.

- Meal 3: 14 points in the protein column, 6 in the vegetable column, 5 in the fruit column, and 4 in the butter and oil column. Here you have plenty of variety. Any meat or fish can fit the 14 points in the protein. And there is infinite variety possible for the rest of the columns.

- Meals 4, 5, and 6: Apply the same substitution principles based on the calopoints available for each column

Debra used this DP template in her own unique way. Her perspective of eating food was a bit different from that of other people. She did not buy into the stereotype of certain foods for breakfast and different foods for dinner. She just liked to eat whatever she wanted whenever she wanted. For example, she sometimes ate oatmeal for dinner. While she consciously made healthy choices, she just fit them into the FDL like a jigsaw puzzle. When the page was done, she was done.

Joyce was a lot more methodical. She would prewrite her entire menu for the day into the FDL immediately after her first meal. Then she simply followed the plan she had set throughout the day.

As you can see, there are many ways to creatively apply the principle of preparation, modifying your eating plan to your preferences. Consider following some of these ideas other people have had and then experiment with a few of your own. Just be sure not to compromise any factor that deviates from the formulas that govern success.

Achieving Consistency in Exercise

Consistent daily exercise is usually a difficult task to accomplish, especially for people who have life schedules that keep changing or who have fluctuations in their daily demands. Obviously, creating a routine by intentionally scheduling the exact time you will dedicate to exercise is ideal, but life is not always that predictable. For that reason you need a Plan B prepared ahead of time to get you back on track if you are derailed by daily demands.

This unpredictability of life is what makes the seventeen- to twenty-minute daily routine done at home so valuable. There is a tendency for a person to stray from the simple basics of their exercise routine to engage in more entertaining activities found at the health club. It is not uncommon for even my most devoted patients to forsake the twenty-minute routine for something more interesting or at least incorporate the exercises into a more elaborate routine at the gym. This is not necessarily negative, except when a problem arises in getting to the gym.

A change in work schedule, a family vacation, or an unforeseen incident can knock a person off their regular exercise routine, especially if it involves a trip to the gym. The next thing you know, you haven't been at the gym in a week and haven't done any exercise at all. That's why it's important to establish an exercise routine that will be unaffected by changing circumstances. Dan's story powerfully illustrates this concept.

Dan joined the program with his sister. He enjoyed sports but was just as satisfied being a spectator as a player. His body fat was over the clinical obesity line; he loved to eat pork buns, which sounded to me like they must contain 1,000 calories apiece. In the beginning, he was kind of aloof in his participation in the program. His sister was very diligent and enjoyed great gains in a short period of time. Dan still logged pork buns on his FDL.

One week I convinced him to give me seven days of the twenty-minute exercise routine plus thirty minutes of running on the treadmill at school. We did a covenant handshake, and I waited for his next week's visit. Happily, Dan had kept his agreement to exercise and was shocked to see he had lost four pounds and 1.5 percent body fat. After that, he became highly motivated, "pysched," to meet his health challenges the next week.

I modified his twenty-minute routine to make it more intense, and he continued his thirty-minute run. In time, he lost forty pounds of fat, added ten pounds of muscle, and got his body fat to 18 percent. Dan was now an athlete. Every day he did his intense twenty-minute routine without fail. On his days off from school, he would go for a run in his neighborhood. The key to his success was the taste of success.

TAKING FULL RESPONSIBILITY

We have discussed the absolute necessity for taking full responsibly for your actions or your lack of appropriate action. Becoming responsible is a critical aspect for completing the program successfully. The people who quit are usually convinced that they are incapable of doing the program because of some extenuating outside circumstance. Those who quit or in some cases never start because of the lack of money or lack of time are not necessarily in this category. Those people have a problem processing their life priorities or believe that one day they will get around to getting into shape when they have more time or their finances are better. The truth is they never do. Some people have to wait for a crisis to occur before they do something about their health. In reality, most people do this; that's why the hospitals are filled to overflowing and the pharmacists dispense millions of prescriptions every day for conditions that can be naturally corrected or avoided if people just took full responsibility for their actions. My hope is that you are not going to be counted as one of those people.

I first met John at a PTA meeting. He was the president of the PTA and was overseeing the event where I was the guest speaker. At the end of the meeting, I heard a big crash. I looked around and saw a crowd gathering around John, trying to pick him up from the floor. At first I was concerned that he had suffered a heart attack. It turns out that John's back, which had been "killing" him all day, just gave out on him, and he fell. He was in tremendous pain and could hardly move.

I went over to the group and proceeded to do what any other "living on the edge" chiropractor would do; I gave him a chiropractic adjustment right there with fifty people watching me. (Talk about a decision that could make or break your practice.) I was not surprised, however, when John got up from the floor in his own strength with a huge smile on his face. I couldn't have written a better ending to my presentation. I breathed a silent thank-you to the Lord for His favor. Immediately John began to thank God that I had been at the meeting. (His thanksgiving was not added to the minutes of the meeting.)

That is how John and his wife, Alma, became patients in my office. I shared some of Alma's story in chapter 4. Because John and Alma were people of faith, it was easy for them to grasp their obligation to respect their body. It was more than an option for feeling good; it was a responsibility of the Christian walk. For many years John had done nothing to improve his physical well-being. He had played football in college, so he knew what it was like to be in shape at one time. Later in life he had suffered several severe injuries that truly became a hindrance to continuing any physical exercise. However, John was not ready to quit.

Over the next several months John and I developed a friendship and trust. I told him every week what he could achieve, and he proved me right. Once in a while the "old" John would show up. The scale would go up, and John would give me the shocked "what just happened, I can't believe it, your scale must be broken, I just weighed myself this morning" routine. He would even try to get his wife in on the justification. When that happened, she would rapidly "sell him down the river." Then we would all laugh, and John would 'fess up to the barbeque chicken and bag of potato chips in which he had indulged. And he would swear that next week would be a better week. The real beauty of his story is that John always took full responsibility and truly kept his word about working harder the next week.

Remember, trying to fool yourself will not bring success. You are in control of your destiny and future as you submit to the Lordship of Christ. You can minimize your chances of contracting preventable diseases if you take full responsibility over the things you can change. Let me reiterate once more my theme verse to emphasize the importance of this biblical principle of ruling over your desires:

> Then God said, "Let Us make man in Our image, according to Our likeness; and let them rule [have dominion] over…"
>
> —GENESIS 1:26

Then consider your answers to these questions:

- Do you think the shape you're in now, inside and out, is the image that God intended for you?

- Do you think the actions you are taking right now concerning your lifestyle habits are reflecting the likeness and attributes of God?

- Are you in a position of dominion and control over your circumstances?

God has designed us, as Christians, to reflect His character and His attributes and to have divine dominion over our environment. The daily task of battling the flesh and exerting dominion over our carnal desires is God's training ground to succeed in that goal. In that way we will prove to the world that we are indeed the expression of Genesis 1:26.

The desire of my heart and the purpose of my Genesis Diet program is to help you attain to the purpose of God for you to give Him glory through your health and wellness. Your obedience to the covenantal principles that govern your health will create a testimony that will surely make you an effective witness for the kingdom of God.

Chapter 12

WHY YOU WILL SUCCEED

T HE HOPE AT this point is to create a permanent change in the way you think, speak, and act about your health and wellness. The strength of your success can be fueled by only two things: your physical desire to live in a vibrant state of well-being and your desire to enjoy life to its fullest. For some readers, this motivation may border on the brink of vanity rather than the promises of God that obedience leads to favor and favor leads to dominion in all your endeavors. However, your desire to be in great shape and to enjoy life to its fullest is by no means based in vanity.

It is true that vanity, which is self-absorbed pride, will always corrupt the internal beauty of a person. On the other hand, humility and submission to the biblical covenants that govern your wellness will always give you the best opportunity to experience optimal wellness. Getting into great shape will also give you a wonderful sense of confidence and let you bring glory to God.

Throughout the Scriptures we read of the unchanging promises of God. The words inspire our hope and optimism that God is on our side, that He will never abandon us, and that our future is filled with favor as we live in submission to the Almighty. However, our continuous interaction with the challenges of daily life, being "in the world" but not "of the world" (John 17:14), can sometimes cause chaos.

There is no book written by man, no lesson taught in school, not even a sermon preached from the pulpit that can teach you how to be safeguarded completely from the evils of this world. Don't be fooled into thinking that someone else has it all together. Even the apostle Paul reminds you that you need to "work out your salvation with fear and trembling" (Phil. 2:12). Whatever else that means, it shows that you must become responsible and accountable to walk in the promises of God for your life. It means that every day is a potential challenge and that you need to turn to the Lord for strength and guidance.

A PERSONAL CHALLENGE

As you prepare to begin your journey to exciting new health goals, I would like to encourage you with these final instructions. First, if you get off track (which is always a possibility), never get disgusted, ashamed, or hopeless. Shake it off and ask God to give you the courage to start again. Even if you have to start several more times, there is no reason to quit. Never judge yourself by another person's progress or standards. Simply read chapters 2 and 3 again and reposition yourself for success. Trust me, you will eventually get it!

Secondly, learn to pray your way through each day's struggles. You will find that prayer will be your most powerful asset to give you strength, put you back on course, and level the mountains of your daily stress. When Jesus taught the disciples to pray what we refer to as the Lord's Prayer, He was really giving us an outline for how to pray (Matt. 6:9–13). For example, He taught us to address our heavenly Father and to hallow His name. We are to ask God for His will on earth (our lives), to be our provider, and to forgive us our trespasses. We ask Him for divine protection from temptation and from evil, and we finish by giving Him honor and glory. As you pray in that way, you will find strength to receive the blessing of God for your life.

In that same way, I thought it would be helpful to give you some guidelines for prayer regarding your establishing a strong foundation for the wellness of your temple. You can use them as your daily confession to empower your thinking by the Author of the spoken word, which creates subsequent actions that lead to success. This kind of prayer can motivate you to achieve greater goals than you would think possible otherwise.

Thank the Lord.

As a believer, you are taught in the Scriptures to begin your conversation with the Lord with thanksgiving for what He has already done for you as your Savior and Lord (Ps. 100:4; Phil. 4:6).

Because God is God, He already knows exactly what you need. Begin with an offering of thanksgiving for carrying you through life to this point. Thank Him for not dealing with you according to your disobedience but in His loving-kindness (Ps. 103:10–11). Thank Him for Christ, who set you on the path for reconciliation and eternal salvation.

Acknowledge your source of wisdom.

Confess your allegiance to the Lord for His leadership. It is very tempting to rely on the advice of others. Pray that the counsel you receive is godly and that the Lord will give you discernment to know the difference.

Regard covenant.

Obedience is the ultimate key to success. God is bound by His Word to bless the obedient. Above all things, ask the Lord to give you wisdom and strength to walk in obedience. That would include being obedient to His covenant for your body as the temple of the Holy Spirit. Pray for the desire to learn more about what you can do to get in shape.

Acknowledge His mercy.

If you have been abusing the mercy of the Lord, you need to take the time to acknowledge His compassion and repent of your ambivalence. Ask the Lord to give you a burning desire to make correct decisions and take correct actions to improve your health, as well as every situation in your life.

Put the Lord first.

There is no corporate crisis intervention manual or airline emergency instruction card or even a first aid kit that carries the instruction: "Before you follow these directions, please seek the Lord God Almighty for advice." On the other hand, the Bible is clear that in all of life we are to seek the Lord first (Matt. 6:33). The New Testament is especially clear in matters of healing that we should pray (James 5). Whenever we sense that we are struggling with obedience, we should stop, seek the counsel of the Lord, and allow the Holy Spirit to empower our obedience.

Acknowledge His creation.

When it comes to the wonder of the design of your physical body, it is easy for the average person to take it for granted. By acknowledging the complex and flawless way God interconnected the physiology of your neurological system with the rest of your body, you recognize God's greatness. It is good to meditate on the wonder that God built innate healing power into your body also. And when faced with the crisis of a serious illness, it is good to confess that you believe God is your Healer as the Scriptures teach.

Protect from the divisiveness of the enemy.

Never underestimate your enemy. Most people are trusting of the people they love, and they also extend that trust to people in authority, especially those who hold the knowledge of sickness and disease. When faced with a health dilemma, be it simple like trying to lose 10 pounds or catastrophic like dealing with the diagnosis of cancer, you should always put into perspective God's point of view. With a simple matter it is easy to take your time and consult God in prayer, but with the more deadly diagnosis the pressure to act swiftly is of paramount urgency. We must remember that the enemy lurks in the shadows of every situation. This does not mean we should be paranoid of every person who gives us health advice or every doctor who gives us a diagnosis and treatment plan. What it does means is we should never leave God out of any decisions we make. If something feels weird in your gut, maybe it's more than just your intuition; maybe it's the prompting of the Holy Spirit. Maybe instead of just listening to your sister the nurse (because she is your sister who happens to be a nurse) or the doctor who has a wall full of plaques, maybe tactfully getting a second opinion will confirm your feeling or reassure your initial recommendations. Either way, always ask the Lord to expose the path that you're a choosing to take.

Ask for discernment.

It is no secret that the world we live in is on information overload. The TV, the radio, magazines, or even a leisurely stroll down Broadway into Times Square turns into an information extravaganza. The biggest culprit when it comes to the distribution of propaganda of health-related information is television and radio broadcasting. Television is filled with pharmaceutical advertisements and "miracle cure" infomercials, while the radio airways are perfect for talk show hosts to promote "breakthrough" products and services. Religious broadcasters are not exempt from promoting what they believe to be valuable health protocols. It is vital that you go to the Lord in prayer, asking for what I like to call "information discernment." You must include in your prayer life the request for discernment of what information is valid and what is a message based in self-gain. Be on guard; the Lord is able to navigate you to the truth. Remember, He taught us to pray, "And lead us not into temptation."

Guard against harboring the enemy.

Earlier I discussed the critical need for walking in forgiveness with others and for eliminating negative emotional sins from your life. According to the Scriptures, this is one of the most critical aspects to be addressed when you are having your conversation with the Lord: "For if you forgive others for their transgressions, your heavenly Father will also forgive you. But if you do not forgive others, then your Father will not forgive your transgressions" (Matt. 6:14–15).

God cannot hear your prayers if you are harboring the attributes of your archenemy, the devil, in your heart. The attributes that the enemy breeds include anger, jealousy, vengeance, unforgiveness, malice, bitterness, spitefulness, manipulation, contempt, and many other nasty characteristics that can fester in your spirit. If you are harboring any of these evil attributes because you were offended or wronged, God cannot operate in an atmosphere that is being tainted by the foul stench of the enemy.

You must ask the Lord to show you if you are harboring any diabolical attitudes and to help you rid yourself of those attributes of the enemy. Choose to forgive, regardless of your feelings, and allow the Lord to cleanse you. That decision will allow the Holy Spirit a place in your heart to create a healing touch and shed His love abroad in your heart (Rom. 5:5).

Rebuke excuses and shortcuts.

In the Lord's Prayer, Jesus taught us to say, "And do not lead us into temptation, but deliver us from evil" (Matt. 6:13). This is a good prayer to pray when you are tempted to take a shortcut regarding your health goals. There will be days that you will undoubtedly like to just stay in bed and pull the covers over your head. You will come up with every old excuse and a few new ones to convince yourself. It is imperative to face these excuses head-on. Don't give them a minute to build momentum. If your flesh is begging you to stay in bed and forget about the exercises, rebuke the thought immediately, pray desperately, and start doing your crunches.

Submit to His will.

It is imperative to submit your will to God. Decisions you make that are not born out of the prompting of the Holy Spirit become ploys of the enemy to try to slow your progress or knock you off course completely. Being willing to be obedient and submissive to the prompting of the Holy Spirit is crucial. In your prayer, declare firmly, "Your will be done" (Matt. 6:10). We all know that working *with* the Lord will always produce a better outcome than working against Him.

Address the past.

There will be times that the enemy will remind you of your past failures and paint a picture of your future tasks as insurmountable mountains. When his accusing voice reminds you of the disappointments of your past, remind him with confidence of the hope and promise of the new day in the Lord's favor. The past can give you advice on how to change your future; never give it the opportunity to *dictate* your future. As for the mountains that lie before you, don't look at the peak from the foothill; always look at the immediate steps upward that your feet are taking. Trust that the Lord has your path to success mapped out one step at a time.

Confess that this is a new day.

Remember the old phrase, "This is the first day of the rest of your life." Every day is a fresh start, a new beginning, and a brand-new opportunity to get things going in the right direction. Take this time to just give thanks that, "This is the day which the LORD has made; let us rejoice and be glad in it" (Ps. 118:24). Confess that this is a new day, and you are going to eat great and do all your exercises. This is the day that you will have no desire for coffee or soda. This is the day that no one will stress you out. This is the day that your chiropractor will give you the perfect adjustment. (This is the one I like for all my patients to confess.) This is the day that you will not allow the enemy to lead you off the path of righteousness.

Be accountable to the King.

Finally, never forget your *ultimate accountability* to the Lord. Remind yourself that the whole reason you're getting into shape, the reason you're choosing a natural path to wellness, is to give Him the honor and glory in your success. You are honoring your obligation as a Christian to respect your body as the temple of the Holy Spirit. You acknowledge that God has a purpose for your life and that He needs you to be happy, healthy, and in a place of good influence to carry out the tasks He has preassigned for your life.

B. J. Palmer, the developer of chiropractic, said, "We never know how far reaching some thing we may think, say, or do, today, will affect the lives of millions tomorrow."[1] This is so true, and this is my hope and prayer for you. I hope that the words of this book have inspired you to think differently about how your body works and the hope that is built into you to heal and enjoy good health. I pray that you speak life into every situation you encounter and that you never allow the enemy to use your tongue to cause harm against yourself or anyone else. And finally that you do what needs to get done, regardless if you like to do it or not, to get yourself into shape for your own good and for the good of those you have influence and persuasion over.

During a four-day seminar in Tulsa, Oklahoma, Dr. Myles Munroe drilled into my head what is now my theme verse:

> Then God said, "Let Us make man in Our image, according to Our likeness; and let them rule over the fish of the sea and over the birds of the sky and over the cattle and over all the earth, and over every creeping thing that creeps on the earth."
>
> —GENESIS 1:26

This scripture is the foundational motivation and inspiration for my work. What good would it be to gain the pleasure of refound health, renewed vitality, and youthfulness; to look great in the mirror and have no fear of an impending disease; and, of course, to add years to your life if in the end you don't acknowledge the God who made this all possible in the first place. Your goal should be to fulfill God's design and plan for mankind to have dominion over all of life.

God has exercised magnificent benevolence in creating you and me in His image and likeness. Through Christ's redemption, we can become the reflection of His character in the earth. He has created a spirit in us that is compatible with His. In mankind He has implanted His attributes and given us ability to access His authority and exercise dominion over life. He has given us the ability and mandate to rule over our environment and even ourselves. Through redemption He has given us complete authority over the enemy (the "creeping thing") who tries tirelessly to separate us from the presence of the King. It is by understanding this awesome divine mandate that I hope you find the strength to complete the task the Lord has assigned you.

If you are a follower of Christ, take a moment to thank Him. If you don't have a personal and intimate relationship with Christ as Savior, take a moment now to ask Christ to be the Lord of your actions and thoughts from now on. God is faithful to hear your cry and give you His wonderful gift of salvation. Then you can count on His help to overcome every obstacle and embrace every attitude for success in living the abundant life He promised. Let me encourage you to enjoy the journey of your Genesis Diet to living a life of optimal wellness as God intended.

Appendix A

FOOD DIARY LOG

Step 1: Determine target calories

Step 2: Record the time of each meal

Step 3: List foods, amounts, and calories

Step 4: Spread meals according to activity

Step 2   **Step 3**

Time	Food Breakdown	C	P	V	F	D	BO	W	E	S
	Goals and totals									

	Total Calories	C	P	V	F	D	BO
	Goals and totals						

Step 4

Step 1

C: Carbohydrates

P: Protein

V: Vegetables

F: Fruit & Berries

D: Dairy

BO: Butter & Oils

W: Water

E: Exercise

S: Supplements

FOOD DIARY LOG

Time	Food Breakdown	C	P	V	F	D	BO	W	E	S
8AM 10%	1 cup of oatmeal	12								
10AM 15%	1 container yogurt, 1 medium apple				5	12				
12N 25%	4 cups mixed salad, 4oz. grilled chicken, grapes		14	6	5		4			
2PM 25%	3 oz. salmon, ½ cup brown rice, 2 cups vegetables	10	12	4			4			
4PM 15%	1 whole wheat bread w/ butter, 3 cups salad	14		2			4			
6PM 10%	almonds and mixed nuts, 3 strawberries		10		2					
	Goals and totals	36	36	12	12	12	12			

Total Calories 1200 or 120 points	Goals and totals	C	P	V	F	D	BO
		30%	30%	10%	10%	10%	10%

Appendix B

TIPS FOR COUNTING CALORIES
IN MIXED FOODS

1. Most boxes, cans, and bags of food will have calorie counts.
   For your goal to be accurate, you need to record the calories
   in the different food groups separately. For example, the
   soup may be a total of 160 calories. Some of the calories are
   carbohydrates from the noodles and vegetables, some are
   protein calories from the chicken, and, of course, they will
   have calories from fat. Though it is far from being exact, you
   can just divide the total calories evenly among these three
   different food groups and record them. Or, if you want to
   play bioengineer, you can apply the science you learned
   in the previous chapter. Carbohydrates and proteins need
   about 4 calories to burn off a gram, while fat needs about 9
   calories to burn off a gram. If your soup contains 12 grams
   of carbohydrates, 12 grams of protein, and 7 grams of fat,
   multiply those numbers by the number of calories needed to
   burn 1 gram of each food group.

2. If you are making a homemade chicken soup for the family,
   you can measure the ingredients to determine calorie count
   or make an educated guess. The object is to keep track of
   all the ingredients. For example, the broth is made from 12
   ounces of chopped-up chicken parts, 2 cups of noodles, 2
   cups of chopped carrots and peas, and ½ cup of chickpeas.
   The total calories are 420 protein calories from the chicken,
   400 carbohydrate calories from the noodles, 40 vegetable calories from the peas and carrots, and 200 more protein calories from the chickpeas, which equals 1,060 calories. If the
   recipe makes 8 cups of soup, each cup would contain 132.5
   calories. You can further break this down if you like, but my
   purpose is not to burden you down with mathematics.

3. On my website I have developed a form I call the "Eat Sheet." This is a simplified guide to the number of calories in specific food sources. You may also refer to Appendix C for a sample Eat Sheet.

4. Finally, there is the reliable Internet. Simply search "calories for pizza," "whole-grain spaghetti," or "vegetable dumplings," for example, and you will get an answer. Also, there are websites, tables, and phone apps and mobile downloads that can instantly give you calorie counts. I have a few patients who have an application on their handheld computer that helps them record the calories of the food they eat in real time.

THE EAT SHEET

ALL THE FOLLOWING amounts are approximate numbers. You should always check the label when you're not sure about the amount and values. Please note the point system below; points are calories minus the last digit (i.e., 200 calories = 20 points).

STARCH GROUP

No more than 30 to 35 percent of points per day

- Pasta and rice/grains, 1 cup cooked – 20 points

- Corn – 14 points

- White potatoes, 1 cup boiled – 15 points; sweet potatoes are slightly lower with a better glycemic index number

- Quinoa, ¼ cup – 15 points

- Whole-wheat bread – 12–15 points per slice

- Bagels – 25–30 points

- Breakfast cereal: always read the label – i.e., Go-Lean Crunch, 19 points

- Oatmeal – 10–15 points per bowl

VEGETABLES

At least 10 percent of points per day; most vegetables are between 10 and 20 calories per cup.

- Lettuce, 2 leaves – 3 calories

- Asparagus – 2 points

- Broccoli – 2 points

- Cabbage (average) – 1 point

- Carrots – 2 points

- Cauliflower – 2 points

- Celery – 1 point

- Cucumber – 1.5 points

- Lettuce (average) – 1 point

- Mushroom – 3 points

- Okra – 1.5 points

- Onion – 1.5 points

- Radish – 2 points

- Spinach – 1–3 points

- Tomatoes – 1–3 points

PROTEIN

Meat, per 4 ounces
No more than 30 to 35 percent of points per day

- Bacon – 50 points

- Beef – 27 points

- Lamb chops, grilled – 36 points

- Lamb leg, roasted – 27 points

- Pork chops, grilled – 34 points

- Veal fillet, roasted – 24 points

- Chicken, grilled – 14 points

- Duck, roasted – 33 points

- Turkey, roasted – 16 points

- Bass, steamed – 12 points

- Catfish, steamed – 10 points

- Cod fillets, baked – 9 points

- Flounder, steamed – 6 points

- Fresh halibut, steamed – 10 points

- Lemon sole, steamed – 8 points

- Salmon, steamed – 18 points

- Tuna – 18 points

Other proteins

- Beans, assorted, ¼ cup – 10 points (no more than 20–40 points per day)

- Egg, hard-boiled – 10 points

- Egg, fried – 12 points

Dairy

Cheese

No more than 15 percent of points per day and taken from the protein group

- American, 1 slice – 10 points

- Blue, 1 slice – 9 points

- Cheddar, 1 slice – 11 points

- Cream cheese, 1 oz. – 10 points

- Cottage cheese, ½ cup – 8 points

- Grated cheese, 1 Tbsp. – 2 points

Other dairy

- Skim milk – 10 points

- Soy milk – 10 points

- Yogurt (read the label) – 10–15 points

Fruit

At least 10 to 15 percent of points per day

- Apple (depending on size) – 5–10 points

- Apricot (depending on size) – 5–10 points

- Orange (depending on size) – 5–10 points

- Peach (depending on size) – 5–10 points

- Pear (depending on size) – 5–10 points

- Plum (depending on size) – 5–10 points

- Melon (depending on size) – 5–10 points

- Kiwi (depending on size) – 5–10 points

- Clementine (depending on size) – 5–10 points

- Nectarine (depending on size) – 5–10 points

- Papaya (depending on size) – 5–10 points

- Mango (depending on size) – 5–10 points

- Grapefruit (depending on size) – 5–10 points

- Pineapple, 1 cup – 5–10 points

- Avocado – 32 points

- Banana – 11 points

- Raspberries, 1 cup – 5 points

- Strawberries, 1 cup – 5 points

- Grapes, 1 cup – 6 points

- Blackberries, 1 cup – 8 points

- Blueberries, 1 cup – 8 points

- Figs, 1 cup – about 10 points

- Prunes, 1 cup – about 10 points

- Raisins, ½ cup – 21 points

- Soy-banana-berry shake – 25 points

Butter and Oils

- Butter, 1 pat – 3.5 points

- Olive oil, 1 Tbsp. – 12 points

- Olives, 5 – 4 points

Miscellaneous Foods

Soups

Most soups, served in 8 oz., are 10 to 16 points. For example, Chicken Asparagus Soup, double portion serving: 4 oz. chopped grilled chicken, 1 bundle diced asparagus, 2 bouillons, 16 oz. water = 18 points.

Pizza

- Cheese pizza, 1 slice – 23 points

- Pepperoni pizza, 1 slice – 29 points

Snack bars

- Zone Bar – 21 points

- Granola bar – 12 points

- South Beach bar – 14 points

Chinese food

- Dim Sims, 1, fried – 10 points

- Spring roll, 1, deep-fried – 11 points

- Wonton, medium, 1, fried – 11 points

- Beef with Chinese vegetables, 1 cup – 25 points

- Lemon chicken – 41 points

- Barbecued boneless ribs, 1 cup – 54 points

- Fried rice, 1 cup – 36 points

- Wonton soup, 1 medium bowl – 24 points

Junk Food

Chips and pretzels

Most potato chips are 15 points per ounce; most pretzels are 10 points per ounce.

Chocolate candy bars

- Kit Kat – 11 points

- Mars – 13 points

- Milky Way – 13 points

- Snickers – 15 points

- Twix – 27 points

Store-bought cookies

- Chocolate chip, 1 cookie – 7 points

- Oreos, 1 cookie – 6 points

Cakes

- 2 oz. slice of cake – 20–30 points

Ice cream

- 8 oz. serving – 30 points

Appendix D

MAKING FOOD SUBSTITUTIONS

- The king of substitutions is to eat whole-wheat, whole-grain, or whole-sprout breads and pastas instead of white breads and regular pasta.

- In addition, you can begin to substitute whole grains for processed grains, such as brown rice instead of white rice. When you visit a health food store, you will see a variety of whole-grain choices such as barley, quinoa, black rice, and, my favorite, spelt. Like the breads, ounce for ounce the whole grains and the white rice are about the same calories, but there is a significant difference in their glycemic indexes. In addition, the whole grains are considerably more nutritious because the husk of the grain (removed from white rice) contains most of the vitamins, mineral, and fiber.

- For chocolate lovers, carob is about half the calories of the same amount of chocolate. With almonds, which are much less caloric and lower in saturated fats than peanuts, you can enjoy an "almond bar."

- If you have to have milk, make a change to low fat or skim milk. If you can switch to almond or soy milk, that may be a healthier choice. However, calorie counts may be the same as cow milk unless you use the low-fat (light) version.

- If you're a bacon and burger lover, try the turkey version. Granted, there is a sacrifice when it come to taste, but giving up a little taste to have less around the waist is not a bad trade off. The turkey versions have a much lower calorie count as well as less saturated heart-stopping fats.

- As for the soda junkies, you are victims of the biggest waste in useless calorie consumption and other unnecessary chemicals. Typical colas are filled with sugar, caffeine, and caramel color. These are non-nutrients we can live without, especially the caffeine, which is often the motivation for drinking soda. In addition, the phosphoric acid and glycerin found in most sodas are harmful. Phosphoric acid is linked to kidney conditions and osteoporosis. (A better use of phosphoric acid is to remove rust from your fence.) To get free from your soda addiction, slowly begin to replace your soda with flavored seltzer and then eventually to flavored water and finally to just plain water.

- For those who love chips and crackers, try switching to low-calorie, low-fat popcorn-based crisps or puffs.

- Keeping your salads low calorie is also important. Salad dressings can be a real killer. Dressings containing oil are especially notorious for tacking on the calories. Even extra-virgin olive oil, in itself very nutritious, still packs 120 calories per tablespoon. If you try balsamic vinegar on your salad a few times, you will forget you ever needed oil in the dressing.

- Switch from coffee to herbal tea. Instead of three cups of coffee a day, make one of the cups herbal tea. The next week make it two cups of tea and one cup of coffee. Eventually make coffee a treat one or two days per week.

- Switch from ice cream to yogurt. Ice cream can be a comfort food to many people, but at 350 totally unhealthy calories a serving, the 90-calorie yogurt can be very convincing. Again, the slow substitution method works wonders.

NOTES

INTRODUCTION

1. Grace Nasri, "Top 10 Overweight U.S. States and Counties," *Huffington Post*, March 21, 2011, http://www.huffingtonpost.com/grace-nasri/america-the-fat-10-counti_b_837358.html#s255309&title=Mississippi_354_percent (accessed August 18, 2011).

2. UPI.com, "U.S. Population: 308,745,538," December 21, 2010, http://www.upi.com/Top_News/US/2010/12/21/US-population-308745538/UPI-94991292951756/ (accessed August 18, 2011).

3. Associated Press, "Obesity Costs U.S. $168 Billion, Study Finds," USAToday.com, October 18, 2010, http://www.usatoday.com/yourlife/fitness/2010-10-18-obesity-costs_N.htm?csp=34news (accessed August 18, 2011).

4. Ibid.

CHAPTER 1

THE *WHY* IS MORE IMPORTANT THAN THE *HOW-TO*

1. *Merriam-Webster's Collegiate Dictionary*, 9th edition (Springfield, MA: Merriam-Webster, Inc., 1983), s.v. "wisdom."

CHAPTER 2

OVERCOMING SPIRITUAL BARRIERS TO YOUR SUCCESS

1. BlueLetterBible.org, "Lexicon Results: Strong's H1285—*Beriyth*," http://www.blueletterbible.org/lang/lexicon/lexicon.cfm?Strongs=H1285t=KJV (accessed August 18, 2011). Also, BlueLetterBible.org, "Search Results for "Covenant" and "G1242," http://www.blueletterbible.org/search/translationResults.cfm?Criteria=covenant%2A+G1242&t=KJV (accessed August 19, 2011).

2. BlueLetterBible.org, "Lexicon Results: Strong's G1653—*Eleeo*," http://www.blueletterbible.org/lang/lexicon/lexicon.cfm?Strongs=G1653&t=KJV (accessed August 19, 2011). Also, BlueLetterBible.org, "Lexicon Results: Strongs' H2617—*Checed*," http://www.blueletterbible.org/lang/lexicon/lexicon.cfm?Strongs=H2617&t=KJV (accessed August 19, 2011).

CHAPTER 5

THE SCIENCE OF LOSING BODY FAT

1. *Merriam-Webster's Collegiate Dictionary*, 10th edition (Springfield, MA: Merriam-Webster, Inc., 1994), s.v. "calorie."

2. Bill Hendrick, "Water May Be Secret Weapon in Weight Loss," WebMD .com, August 23, 2010, http://www.webmd.com/diet/news/20100823/water-may-be-a-secret-weapon-in-weight-loss (accessed August 22, 2011).

3. Michael J. Breus, "Sleep Habits: More Important Than You Think," WebMD.com, March 15, 2006 http://www.webmd.com/sleep-disorders/guide/important-sleep-habits (accessed August 22, 2011).

CHAPTER 6

THE GENESIS DIET AND EXERCISE PROGRAM

1. Mayo Clinic staff, "Counting Calories: Get Back to Weight-Loss Basics," December 19, 2009, http://www.mayoclinic.com/health/calories/WT00011 (accessed August 22, 2011).

CHAPTER 10

ELIMINATING THE STRESS FACTOR

1. Ira Levin, *The Stepford Wives* (n.p.: Fawcett Crest, 1973).

CHAPTER 11

THE EXPERIENCE OF OTHERS

1. ThinkExist.com, "Bobby Unser Quotes," http://thinkexist.com/quotation/success_is_where_preparation_and_opportunity_meet/200903.html (accessed August 26, 2011).

CHAPTER 12

WHY YOU WILL SUCCEED

1. B. J. Palmer, *The Philosophy of Chiropractic* (n.p.: 1920), chapter 4, "Truth," as quoted in Gary Farr, "The Wisdom of B. J. Palmer," April 17, 2002, http://www .becomehealthynow.com/article/chirohistory/590/ (accessed August 29, 2011).

JOIN THE
GENESIS LIFE
www.schoolofwellness.com

Featuring the
GENESIS LIFE
7 WEEKS TO WELLNESS PROGRAM
Our exclusive online video training program designed
to get you in the best shape of your life. The program
includes dozens of video lessons and demonstrations all
from a biblical perspective.

"SPECIAL BONUS"
The GEN-Intensity Workout
This is our elite 7 week high-intensity workout
for those who dare to take their fitness level from
"good" to "great."

Don't forget to just visit the website at:
www.schoolofwellness.com
and check out all the FREE RESOURCES
just for being a GENESIS DIET student.